ABOUT THE AUTHOR

Dr Ken Goss (DClinPsy) is a consultant clinical psychologist. He was Head of Service/Lead Psychologist for Adult Eating Disorders in Coventry and Warwickshire, UK, from 2001 to 2024. He provides training nationally and internationally, offers clinical supervision, and offers consultation on service development and delivery.

In his early clinical career, he was trained and supervised by Professor Paul Gilbert, the originator of compassion focused therapy (CFT). He is a founding member of The Compassionate Mind Foundation.

He has more than thirty years' experience of working with people with eating disorders and eating distress. He pioneered the development of compassion focused therapy for this population (CFT-E). He is the author of *The Compassionate Mind Approach to Beating Overeating*, the first book to apply CFT to people who struggle with eating distress.

Also by Dr Ken Goss

The Compassionate Mind Approach to Beating Overeating

THE EATING WELL WORKBOOK

WORKBOOK

Addressing Overeating
Using Your Compassionate Mind

DR KEN GOSS

ROBINSON

ROBINSON

First published in Great Britain in 2025 by Robinson

1 3 5 7 9 10 8 6 4 2

Copyright © Dr Ken Goss, 2025
Illustrations by Liane Payne

The moral right of the author has been asserted.

Important Note
This book is not intended as a substitute for medical advice or treatment.
Any person with a condition requiring medical attention should consult
a qualified medical practitioner or suitable therapist.

A CIP catalogue record for this book is available from the British Library.

ISBN: 978-1-47214-760-8

Typeset in Palatino by Initial Typesetting Services, Edinburgh
Printed and bound in Great Britain by Clays Ltd, Elcograf S.p.A.

Papers used by Robinson are from well-managed forests
and other responsible sources.

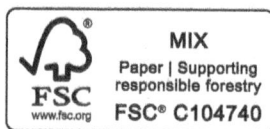

MIX
Paper | Supporting
responsible forestry
FSC www.fsc.org
FSC® C104740

Robinson
An imprint of
Little, Brown Book Group
Carmelite House
50 Victoria Embankment
London EC4Y 0DZ

The authorised representative
in the EEA is
Hachette Ireland
8 Castlecourt Centre
Dublin 15, D15 XTP3, Ireland
(email: info@hbgi.ie)

An Hachette UK Company
www.hachette.co.uk

www.littlebrown.co.uk

Contents

Acknowledgements

My first thanks go to all those clients who have been willing to share their experience of eating disorders, eating distress and overeating. Their insights have been invaluable, while their courage and commitment to learning ways to deal with their experiences and feelings have inspired my work for over thirty years.

This book would never have been written without the support and encouragement of Professor Paul Gilbert. I have had the privilege of working with Paul for almost my entire professional career. His influence has been profound in both my personal and my professional life. He has pioneered the development of compassion focused therapy, and his commitment to developing, researching and promoting this approach has moved compassion into the mainstream of scientific thinking and clinical practice. I will always remain grateful for his help, and for encouraging me to take responsibility for bringing the developments I have made in working with people with eating disorders, eating distress and overeating to a wider audience.

A big thank you to Andrew McAleer and the editorial team at Robinson Psychology for their endless patience and enthusiasm in editing the various iterations of this book – without them it would make a lot less sense!

Another big thank you to Dr Lesley Armitage, who has pioneered using a compassion focused approach via guided self-help for people who overeat. She has helped fine-tune many of the chapters in the book and has led on writing the clinician's guide to this workbook.

I would like to thank my family – Gill, Adam and Tasha – for their support, encouragement and wisdom. I feel blessed and proud to be part of their world. It is my greatest hope that they will always experience compassion from others, offer it to themselves and continue to put it back into the world.

Finally, I would like to thank you, the reader, for taking the time to consider developing a new relationship with food, one that focuses on your physical and psychological wellbeing. I hope it can help you to find new ways to care for yourself and manage the challenges of life.

1 Introduction

Thank you so much for picking up this book. I hope it will be part of your journey to developing a more compassionate relationship with your mind and body, particularly if you, like so many others, have difficulties with overeating.

I am a consultant clinical psychologist, researcher, trainer and supervisor, with over thirty years' experience of working with people with an eating disorder. I developed a compassion focused approach to eating disorders (CFT-E) with the guidance, support and encouragement of my mentor (and good friend) Professor Paul Gilbert. He developed compassion focused therapy to help people experiencing difficulties with shame and self-criticism, and I was lucky enough to be with him at the beginning of that journey. Compassion focused therapy is now used in clinical settings for people with a range of mental health and physical health difficulties and is also used to improve psychological wellbeing for the wider public (for example, in schools and businesses). From small beginnings over twenty-five years ago, I am proud to say that CFT-E is now widely used by eating disorder services in the UK and around the world.

For many years I have been interested in the similarities between those people I see as clients in a mental health setting and those who struggle with overeating in the community. I have also been saddened and angered by the way people who overeat are often portrayed in the media (as lazy and lacking self-discipline) or offered 'quick fixes' by a diet industry that knows the vast majority of people will lose some weight, only to regain it (or put on even more weight) at the end of each dieting cycle. The cost of this in human terms is huge, with many people experiencing shame and self-criticism when a diet does not work. I am also angry about the lack of services or support that would help address this from a scientific, evidence-based approach. Research suggests that there are many similarities between the people I see in clinic and the people I have written this book for. Professor Gilbert wisely advised me to focus my anger into doing something that might be helpful, and that advice began my journey to writing this book and hopefully doing my small part to address these issues.

How to use this book

This book will help you think about the common difficulties with eating that all humans have, and it will help you to explore and change your personal relationship with food, eating and your body.

You should make time for yourself to use the book. Each chapter has questions and exercises to help you understand how and why you eat and learn ways to change your relationship with food and your body. You may find it useful to keep notes or a journal of your thoughts and feelings about the things you read or the exercises you are doing. You may choose for this to be a private journey, or you might want to share this work with a supportive friend or with a professional. I have included details of voluntary and professional organisations in the 'Useful resources' section, if you choose this path. The book also contains reflections and feedback from others who have used these methods themselves.

This book consists of two intertwined elements: an outline of the compassionate mind approach to human psychology, and specifically to our relationships with food, eating and our bodies; and a practical programme of staged tasks that will enable you to relate these ideas to your own life and your own habits, thoughts and feelings around food and eating. You will find exercises you can do and worksheets you can use to keep records. Try these in your own time and at your own pace. Blank copies of the various worksheets can be found at overcoming.co.uk/715/resources-to-download. You can print as many of these as you need – and you may wish to adapt them to make them personal to you. As mentioned previously, you may also find it useful to have a notebook and pen with you as you work through the book so that you can make your own notes on things that you find particularly useful or challenging.

This book contains a lot of ideas, and on first reading it may seem to you that the prospect of change is too complex, difficult or overwhelming. The key is to go one step at a time: try things out for yourself, see what you can use, and if you only change one or two things, that's still helpful.

Understanding our relationship with food

Food can be a pleasure or a curse. Without it we die, and with too much we develop a whole range of health problems. We eat because we're hungry, to be sociable, because we're miserable, or because we just like the taste and the pleasure of putting things in our mouth. We enjoy our food because of its tastes and textures. For most of us, chocolate cake and ice cream are an awful lot more desirable than turnips and spinach. Unfortunately, the latter are much better for us. Although over half the world does not have enough to eat, many of us have the opposite problem – managing the availability of relatively cheap and appetising food. The abundance of easily accessible processed foods brings with it serious difficulties relating to our desire for food and our appetites and weight. In the modern Western world, we are surrounded with enticements to buy and eat more. If we follow these cultural demands, we are pretty likely to put on weight but then become the target of moral and medical condemnation, feeling guilty or ashamed about our eating. Simply telling ourselves not to eat too much is no help. Indeed, it tends to make things worse because we now feel depressed, so we eat more to feel better. Sometimes it can feel as if you just can't win!

What does a 'compassionate mind' approach mean?

When we look more closely at overeating, we come to understand how complex it is, and to realise that it's not our fault that so many of us struggle to regulate our eating behaviour and weight. Our brains have evolved to be attracted to foods that are high in fat and sugar, and our bodies have evolved to store excess energy (in the form of fat) for leaner times. Your brain is not really designed to regulate eating, because for much of the time over which mammals have evolved it didn't need to: we had to make the most of it when it was available.

Once we give up blaming ourselves for the problems we have with our diets and our weight, we become less ashamed and more open to taking responsibility for finding ways to eat, and to exercise, that are appropriate and helpful for us. This is a hard task, and it's even more difficult to tackle it if we are swamped by self-critical feelings.

A compassionate mind approach starts with understanding what we're up against. This means understanding how, and in what conditions, our brains evolved to give us certain desires and passions, and how modern environments can make life both easier for us in some ways and very difficult in others.

Understanding the problem: why we love to eat

Let's go back a million years or so and consider how our ancestors lived. They would have spent much of their time foraging, because food was usually in short supply and they were not as good at hunting as other meat-eating animals such as lions, wolves and hyenas. Foraging animals eat as often as they can because food is often hard to find. Seeking it out requires time and energy, and foragers are constantly on the move. In this environment, our brains did not evolve mechanisms for self-restraint because they did not need them; we evolved for the 'see food' diet: 'see food and eat it'! You may recognise the same tendency in your family dog. It's not our fault that our brains and bodies did not evolve with effective mechanisms for self-restraint in eating, but this can make life very difficult for us in the modern world, where many of us have easy access to cheap, nutritious food and tend to be far less active than our pre-industrial ancestors.

What about the food itself? Well, most of the food our ancestors would have foraged for would have been pretty low in calories, and so they needed to eat a lot of it. We also became hunters of meat and could bring down large game, particularly when we operated in teams. However, hunting tends to be a hit-and-miss affair: even the most successful carnivores actually make a meal out of only about one in ten of their intended prey. So, although meat and fish was an important part of our ancestors' diet, it was a bonus; for the most part they would have relied on foods that could be gathered: nuts, berries, root vegetables and other plants.

Many plants evolved fruits and seeds that were palatable to herbivores, so that they would eat them and spread the seeds; thus, when ripe, they were sweet tasting, as a result of a high sugar content that made them both appetising and naturally high in calorie (energy) content. In fact, the sugary taste is how we know they are ripe: plants that are poisonous or not ripe tend to have a sour taste. Therefore, we evolved with a sweet tooth!

Other energy-dense foods (such as fish or meat) tend to have higher fat and protein contents. They were harder for hunters to obtain but they keep us fuller for longer, which gave hunters an evolutionary advantage in times of famine. In more bountiful times it also meant that, rather than having to constantly forage, humans had time for thinking and making things. This led to an explosion in human development, as we became toolmakers and planners.

However, as these high-fat and high-sugar foods were in short supply, we never had to develop the means to restrain our appetites or our weight – we simply didn't need a brain that would do this! The trouble is that now (for those fortunate to have access to cheap and nutritious food), the see-food-and-eat-it brain is no longer helpful. Indeed, it is becoming a major problem for many of us, who are eating much more than our ancestors and taking far less exercise, developing unhealthy eating habits and becoming overweight as a result.

To make matters worse, we also evolved to be an energy-conserving species. This means that when we have eaten enough to meet our energy needs, we will tend to become less active. We only get more active when we need to go and find more food because we are hungry. So, we have an inherent tendency to become couch potatoes!

There is another interesting aspect to our story. We know that the process of human evolution began around two million years ago, and, along the way, we became a strongly cooperative species, wanting to share a whole range of resources and information with one another. Indeed, language would not have evolved had we not taken an interest in communicating with each other. Hunting relied on social cooperation and the subsequent sharing of the meal. The most successful hunters (those lions, wolves and hyenas) are very sociable within their own groups; they follow very specific rules about eating after a kill to ensure that those who are most valuable to the group all receive a share. We think that these habits also developed among our human ancestors, and so getting food and sharing it became strongly linked to our social lives. Even today, one of the most important ways we entertain others is to cook for them, and we love going out for meals together.

Being fed has always been a comforting experience for humans. Breastfeeding has calmed babies the world over for millennia. Feeding can be soothing – understandably, as it signals the physical closeness of a caregiver and the safeness that this offers. Eating in social groups has also been with us for thousands of years; and still today, eating together and sharing our food solidifies our relationships. Where resources are scarce, it helps us manage their use effectively. When they are more plentiful, we want to share high-quality food, to be seen as generous and as good cooks. Thus, eating together can be a source of both pleasure and social comfort. So, there is nothing wrong with deriving comfort from food. However, at most times in human history the comfort derived from food was self-limiting: mothers can only produce so much milk, and social groups often struggled to find enough to eat.

Our natural preference for sweet foods can easily be used to train us to behave in certain ways, and such foods may soothe us (as we will explore in Chapter 3). The link between them and approval – 'being a good boy or girl' – is made early if sweets are given as a reward for behaving in a particular way. For example, imagine you are in a crowded supermarket, your child is crying, and you know you will be stuck in the queue for at least another twenty minutes. It is easy to see how we could end up giving them a sweet, both to take their mind off their distress and to comfort them, and of course parents learn that it can work! So, they do it again and again. So, what do we do when we are upset as adults? We do what we have learned to do, of course – where's that chocolate? What do we do when we feel we want a reward or want to celebrate? Go for the food and drink, the good night out or a raid on the fridge. We sometimes find that people with eating problems as adults were often soothed with food as children, rather than with hugs or by talking things through and learning how to manage emotions. Indeed, some people are not aware of the link between their emotions and eating.

Of course, until recently in most parts of the world, cakes, chocolate bars, chips and crisps weren't available to be used as treats and pacifiers. But today, from the day we are born to the day we die, food is linked in our minds to enjoyment, treats, celebrating, socialising, having friends, caring, calming difficult emotions and a sense of deserving – and much more. It is unlikely that there has been any time in our history where food has had such complex and multiple associations and meanings.

In a world in which we all have less and less time to care for ourselves and others, where many of us are working in two or more jobs just to keep up, food (and of course drink) has become one way in which we have learned to reward ourselves, manage our feelings or comfort those around us. It's not surprising, then, that those of us who have grown up in the past century have increasingly associated food with comfort and soothing of distress on the one hand, and with rewards and having a good time on the other.

We must be honest, too, in acknowledging that sometimes our problems with food relate to quite complicated emotional difficulties. We know that some children are relatively neglected or come from difficult and abusive families. Having never really felt loved or connected or worthy, they can spend a lot of time as adults trying to cope with difficult emotions with roots in their childhoods. Food can get caught up in all that. Someone who tended to binge-eat once told me that it was like a rebellion: she could do it, and no one could stop her. It was also a way of keeping down painful feelings which at times came close to overwhelming her. 'Food,' she said, 'thinking about it, imagining it, planning to eat and enjoying it – is a way of distracting myself. Problem is, after I finish bingeing, I feel disgusted with myself and so the whole cycle starts up again, fuelled by anger that I can't do anything about.'

Some people struggling to cope with emotional difficulties in this way develop serious eating disorders such as bulimia or anorexia. These are usually best tackled with professional support, though self-help certainly can have a part to play. However, many people who do not develop these grave illnesses still struggle with their eating habits, and often feel angry, ashamed and anxious, habitually binge-eat, raid the fridge when they are upset or find it hard to stop eating once they have started. If any of these descriptions ring a bell and you want to develop a healthy relationship with food in a way that will care for your physical and emotional needs, then this book is for you.

It is important to recognise and have compassion for the complexity of our relationship with food, eating and weight. If we are gentle with and kind to ourselves, if we accept this complexity and the pain that can be hidden behind the 'food problem', we have a better chance of working with these issues. All the time keep in mind that if you're struggling with food there are reasons for it that are to do with how all humans have evolved, which is hardly something you can blame yourself for! Once you come to understand this, and then free yourself from the shame and the blame that so often go with overeating, you can then move on to think about what's really going to help you; what's really in your best interests and how you can look after and urge yourself on to be your very best – and yes, you do deserve that, even if a little voice in your head says, 'Oh no you don't.'

The perils of modern societies and supermarkets

As the human brain evolved, so did its intelligence, and it wasn't far along the road of human evolution that we worked out that you don't need to look for food – you can make it come to you. Humans became farmers, planting crops rather than going out to gather them, and herding and breeding livestock rather than roaming the plains looking for animals to kill. No longer did we have to spend our time firing arrows that missed the buffalo by a mile and getting back to camp exhausted; we simply went to the pen and knocked one on the head. It wasn't quite a supermarket yet, but we were on our way. Over time, of course, barter and then money came into the equation and food became a commodity to be traded like many others – and so, over the past few thousand years, we have trudged down the trail towards modern capitalist societies where we get our food in a totally different way from how we evolved to find and eat it. It's all much easier, of course, but it's created new problems.

Modern Western societies have allowed industries to exploit that old evolutionary 'see-food-and-eat-it' drive in our brains, and those deep and powerful associations between food, pleasure and security. The food industry spends billions artificially enhancing the taste, texture and look of foods to tempt us to buy them and to associate them in our minds with having a good time, surrounded by happy people. Sometimes foods are advertised as 'secret pleasures', but usually the subliminal message is that eating high-fat and high-sugar foods goes with social pleasures such as enjoying family outings or parties.

Not only are the foods themselves tempting but the ways in which they are packaged and displayed are designed to tempt you even more. Supermarkets employ psychologists to help them find the most effective ways to do this. For example, that smell of freshly baked bread stimulates your appetite, and the sight of the cream cakes and two-for-one offers encourages you to buy more than you might have planned. Sweets are placed near checkout tills where stressed shoppers, accompanied by bored children, can easily reach them.

Of course, this isn't to cast supermarkets as out-and-out villains: they're not deliberately trying to cause problems, and they also provide us with good-quality fresh food, including a wide range of fruit and vegetables that even a few years ago were not readily available to most people. However, they're not in business to help us manage our eating either. Instead, they provide what we are prepared to buy and entice us to buy and consume as much of it as we will pay for, and we evolved to prefer sweet and fatty foods.

Modern societies have a rather damaging tendency to blame the individual for problems that are in fact side effects of our new ways of living, and to see them as our individual, rather than collective, responsibility to sort out. But it's really difficult for most of us to understand how our brains and bodies, which evolved in a very different environment over many thousands of years, are responding to demands and enticements that have come into being over mere decades. So, rather than seeing the problem clearly, we get squeezed in the middle between the pressures to overeat and the warnings that we shouldn't. As a result, we end up feeling inadequate, ashamed, helpless and hopeless in managing our eating and weight. So, it is not surprising that we turn to the diet industry for ready-made answers and then blame ourselves when these solutions do not work.

Our need for compassion

It doesn't take long to begin to understand the problems we face and to see that we are dealing with complex relationships between our current diets, our weight and our feelings about ourselves. We may eat because we are happy, because we're just enjoying eating or because we're celebrating (speaking personally, feel-good times are actually my danger times). We may eat because everybody else is and we just go along with that. We may eat because we feel miserable and alone or to distract us from the unhappiness and difficulties in our lives.

Our compassionate journey towards a healthy relationship with food must begin with a clear understanding that this relationship is a complex one. The way our brains have evolved has set us up to have problems that our modern society has simply added to – and that we're not responsible for either! The moment you begin to move away from self-blaming and self-criticism, to take shame out of the complicated web of feelings associated with eating, you will be free to think about how to help yourself in a more compassionate and responsible way. Rather than fighting against temptations, you can learn to work with them.

The key message of this book, then, is this: your overeating is not your fault, but you can take responsibility for and gain control over it if you are supportive and compassionate to yourself along the way. As the book progresses – and particularly in Chapter 4 – we will investigate more thoroughly what being compassionate to yourself means. An advert on television may tell you that being nice to yourself is treating yourself to boxes of chocolates – but if you eat too many, you may be giving yourself health problems. It's much more compassionate to learn how to acknowledge and respond to your real needs, rather than being easy prey to tempters who really just want you to spend money on their products!

Physical and psychological health professionals, too, need to understand this message very clearly. I see many clients who tell me that their conversations with professionals have left them feeling rather ashamed and criticised. There has been an undertone that being overweight is simply about greed or laziness, about lack of willpower, control, or effort – well, lack of everything, really. Having been shamed, blamed and stigmatised, of course people simply turn off, tune out, get depressed, withdraw and take solace in the only thing that can be guaranteed to give them a little pleasure – food! They may also feel a certain amount of anger and rebelliousness – one person who had been told off by a professional went back home and thought, 'How rude you are – how unkind – and how much you don't understand me – well, to hell with you, then', and raided the fridge.

Moving away from moral judgements about eating

Most of us who overeat will diet at some point to manage our weight or our appetite for certain foods. All weight-loss diets aim to restrict our eating below the level of energy that our body needs, but we may also try to limit the types of food we eat because they are seen as in some way unhealthy. For example, until relatively recently diabetics were required to cut out all sugary foods to manage their condition (these rules have been relaxed as the medical profession has recognised that such a restrictive diet is not usually necessary and that clients find it very difficult to maintain anyway).

Anyone who has tried to diet will be only too well aware that television programmes, magazines and diet books are full of conflicting advice and pseudoscience. The diet industry is worth billions worldwide, and hardly a month goes by without some new fad or diet being launched, or some celebrity telling us how they lost 5 kilograms in a week! And yet, despite all this advice, the Western world is plagued by obesity and related diseases, by eating disorders and eating problems – some of which can have profound psychological and physical consequences. With so many conflicting messages, we can feel damned if we diet and damned if we don't.

Many of these diets also contain hidden messages – for example, that if you have a weight problem then it's because there is some-thing wrong with you. They imply that if you are a reasonable person you will want to lose weight by controlling your eating; so, if you don't, then somehow you must be an unreasonable or weak-willed person. A lot of diets also imply that with a little willpower – and, of course, their diet – controlling your eating and losing weight is really not so difficult. Therefore, if you're finding it tough going, if you have a few successes but then put the weight back on again, that is again because there's a problem with you. No wonder many people who are overweight or strug-gling with their eating feel ashamed!

There are even competitive reality TV programmes that follow people as they struggle to manage their weight. These entice us to pass judgement on those who are succeeding or failing in their battle with food and the scales. These programmes feed – and feed on – our fascination with people's struggles but also invite us to treat those 'contestants' who don't make it at best dismissively and, at worst, with contempt and ridicule. We are not encouraged to feel sympathy or understand the complex reasons for their relationship with food and their bodies, to hear of (maybe) the stories of early emotional neglect or the sadness and loneliness of a bullied childhood. Nor are we invited to follow the longer-term journey that these people take – including those who 'win' but regain weight later.

Current evidence suggests that only one dieter in twenty who loses a significant amount of weight will maintain the loss in the long term. Even people taking part in research trials, with a high degree of professional support, are unlikely to lose more than 4–10 kilograms and maintain this for at least a year. If we are overweight, only a moderate amount of weight loss (approximately 5–10 per cent) is necessary to provide some improvement in health, and anything more than this tends to be impossible to maintain. Yet most diet programmes promote a far higher level of weight loss than this and suggest that the results can be maintained for ever if only we follow their advice.

Of course, anyone who has ever been on a diet (and that includes me) will know that losing weight, and keeping it off, is pretty tricky. However, when we run into obstacles it is common for us to blame ourselves, and this tendency is supported by many diet regimes. For example, negative attitudes and moral judgements about food and eating are often reflected in the language used: certain foods are seen as a 'sin' or a 'treat'; or are given 'points', values that are to be earned. Being weighed in front of others at a slimming club can be seen as a supportive gesture, but also as a way of putting pressure on participants through the potential for ritual humiliation in front of the group. Many of these diets and clubs focus on successes with weight loss, holding them up as positive motivation – but what about those who feel too ashamed to reach out for help, or who wander off because they feel they are failing?

I work with many people who have come to see eating as bad, or a sin, or something they have to earn, rather than something their body needs to do in order to function; people who report binge-eating after being weighed publicly, either as a treat for their success or as a punishment for not losing enough. A compassionate mind approach needs to move away from these moral judgements and their inherent criticism of our need and desire to eat. It requires us to support the changes we wish to make without attacking ourselves when we struggle, as we inevitably will. We also need to learn to focus more on our health and wellbeing and less on the feelings of competition that can be associated with seeing the numbers on the scales go down, and to learn other ways to feel a sense of success and to be comforted when we are distressed. This means putting food back in its place, as an important and enjoyable part of our lives, something that can be shared with others, and not a threat to our health or sense of personal wellbeing.

It is likely that your mind will come up with many fears, blocks and resistances along the way. It is important to make a note of these, and we will work on ways to address them throughout the book. These are perfectly normal, as you may have thought for a long time that your current approach to dieting and eating would be helpful for you. A client once said that 'The idea of developing self-compassion feels hard. I want to care for myself, but I don't have enough time for myself. I care for everyone else. I tend to just get on with it.' They had to work on when and how they could find time for themselves and have the courage to prioritise their own needs for short periods during the day. The self-compassion exercises in the book helped them to do this.

Sometimes we decide that we are not going to engage with old coping behaviours, or we want to understand the causes of our suffering, but do not feel that we can tolerate our distress. At these times, knowing that we have a way to alleviate our distress can be very helpful. It can give us the courage to understand why we became distressed and learn new ways to cope. In this book we will work on developing new ways to manage your emotions and to care for yourself more compassionately.

Managing distress

Often when we are distressed it is hard to think about what we can do or who can help us. It may be that there are people who you can talk to directly to manage your distress, or who don't know anything about your difficulties but can provide a helpful temporary distraction from the things that are upsetting you, or remind you that there are people who do care about you and want to spend time with you. It can also be helpful to have a distress management plan that you can turn to if needed. You may wish to complete Worksheet 1 and keep a copy with you (e.g. on your phone) so that you always have it available if you need it. You can find a list of some websites to help you in the 'Useful resources' section at the back of the book.

Worksheet 1: Who can help me if I am distressed?

Friends/family	Name	Contact details
Voluntary agencies	Name	Contact details
Professionals	(e.g. my doctor)	

How this book works

In this book we will explore some of the contradictions involved in trying to change our weight, and some of the obstacles we may meet. This will include looking at how our bodies have evolved to eat and drink and regulate our appetite. We will also look at how our body manages our attempts to eat too much or too little food. We will see how, if we attempt to alter our natural mechanisms, this can have a significant effect on our ability to let our body maintain its weight. We will explore how to find out what our personal healthy weight is – and this doesn't mean an 'ideal weight' according to weight charts and diet books, but one that is ideal for us to function healthily.

I hope that as you read through this book you will find ways to get back in touch with your body. You will learn to respond to the need for food and drink, and to manage some of the complex challenges that our new ways of producing and consuming food pose to letting us reach our naturally healthy weight. As you discover more about the complex links between food and our emotional life, and find ways to disentangle the two, you can let your body do what it is designed to do (stay healthy) and find other ways to manage your thoughts and feelings instead of using food to do this.

Self-criticism is incredibly common in people who diet. This is often one of the most important factors in lowering our mood and isolating ourselves. Moreover, constant self-criticism when our diets don't work, or when we break the rules we set around what, when and how we should eat, is almost bound to lead to failure in our attempts to manage our eating. The new understandings and skills you will learn in this book will help you develop a new relationship with food and eating, free you from unhelpful self-criticism, and increase your chance of letting your body find a weight that is healthy and sustainable for you. You might like to think about whether you tend to criticise yourself a lot, particularly around issues of size, shape, weight and eating. If you do, then this book is probably going to be useful to you.

The key to the approach set out in this book is learning to be compassionate towards ourselves and others. Compassion begins with understanding, and the early chapters aim to help you come to a better understanding of how our brains and bodies work. This is not another diet book, although it will help you find ways to manage your food intake and energy output that are more in tune with your body's needs. Instead, it offers you a different approach to learning to live in a complex body, in a world it is not evolved to live in, with a mind that also hasn't really evolved to deal with all these problems in the first place! It could help you find new ways to deal with the very complex challenges we all face as human beings, particularly in a rich country where food is plentiful. These challenges include:

- to learn to regulate our eating in a way that is best for both our physical health and psychological wellbeing

- to be able to accept and live comfortably with the notion that there are normal variations in human size, shape and weight, and that the shape we might wish to be might not be the size or shape we are biologically designed to be

- to be able to accept and value human beings, including ourselves, regardless of weight and shape

- to be able to manage our feelings without using food as our main or only way of coping with distress.

Most of the chapters contain exercises to help you explore these issues. You may well come to think, as I have, that our bodies are pretty tricky things and that managing them can be hard work; but I hope you will also come to believe that it is possible to do so – without constantly criticising ourselves or feeling under pressure, and without 'going on a diet'. We will explore a different approach that involves learning to respond to our body's needs. This is more likely to lead to long-term weight change and stability than following any of the myriad dietary fads that, although initially appealing, usually end in failure.

In Chapter 2, we explore our relationship with food and eating. It introduces 'set point theory': the idea that your body evolved to keep you at a healthy weight if you feed it enough energy on a regular basis. We will also explore the various ways in which you can affect your body's 'set point', including eating too much or too little, your eating pattern, other substances you take into your body, and of course your emotional life.

In Chapter 3, we will explore the complex relationship between eating and our emotions and thoughts. It introduces the 'three systems' (or circles) model of emotional regulation. We will also examine the impact that dieting, or denying ourselves foods, can have on our feelings, and how this in turn can lead us to feeling self-critical and ashamed.

In Chapter 4, we will explore the meaning of compassion in relation both to our attitudes to food and to our overall emotional wellbeing. We will explore some of the mindsets that lead us to overeat and consider how a more compassionate mindset can help us manage life's challenges in a more effective way.

In Chapter 5, we help to prepare our minds for compassion. It includes exercises to learn to focus our attention, become more mindful and calm our mind and body by deliberately turning on our soothing system.

We expand on these skills in Chapter 6, concentrating on developing our compassionate mind. We will explore new ways of thinking and acting from a self-compassionate perspective that can help you move away from the mindsets and patterns of behaviour that so often lead to overeating.

Chapter 7 explores some of the common fears, blocks and resistances people can have to developing a compassionate approach. Many people find this difficult but, as we will see, through gentle practice and persistence we can train our minds to work in this different way.

In Chapter 8, we explore how to address difficult thoughts and feelings. It provides ways to manage in the short term by using distraction techniques, tolerating distress for long enough to learn what we need to do about it in the longer term, and using our compassionate mind to help us through compassionate thought balancing or letter writing.

In the later chapters, we will work on understanding how your overeating has developed and what keeps it going now. Chapter 9 introduces diary-keeping to help you make sense of your current eating patterns and triggers. Chapter 10 outlines the compassionate mind approach to understanding the influences on your overeating, including the key threats it may have helped you to deal with, and how the unintended consequences may have made you likely to carry on overeating. Chapter 11 brings all this together to help you develop your own personal 'formulation' of how overeating works for you, so that you can use it as a basis for helping resolve overeating for good.

We begin Chapter 12 by looking at the process that we all go through, in one way or another, when making changes in our lives, and how this is likely to affect you when tackling overeating. It also provides exercises to help you explore, maintain and increase your motivation to address overeating and improve your overall wellbeing, and to help you manage setbacks with compassion.

In Chapter 13, we explore how to work out what your body needs in terms of energy and nutrition, so that you can use this as a basis for changing your eating. In Chapter 14, we outline the steps to a healthy relationship with food and eating based on and maintained with compassion, starting with eating more regularly and managing foods that can trigger overeating. In Chapter 15, we build upon this foundation to help you plan to meet your nutritional needs, as you learn to recognise and respond to feeling hungry and full, to care for your body – and, finally, to enjoy eating!

Chapter 16 sets out a summary of the key points of this approach. At the end is a section of 'Useful resources' that may be valuable as you work through the book, and in the future.

I have used examples of several clients in the book. These are fictitious characters, but their histories and the problems they face are typical of many people I have worked with. None of them is based on any particular person, but they have been developed to help you explore particular mindsets that can drive overeating.

This book is designed for most of us who overeat, and many people will be able to work through it happily and productively on their own. You may, however, find that you want some more support. I have written the book with this in mind, so that you can also use it with the help of a friend or in collaboration with a professional therapist. Also, if you are pregnant or have a serious physical illness it would be a good idea to consult a physician or dietitian, as the broad guidelines about your energy needs may not be specific enough for your particular needs. Dr Lesley Armitage and I have also developed a clinician's guide for professionals who are using this book to help people who need additional support to make changes in their relationship with food. It is available to download free of charge from overcoming. co.uk/715/resources-to-download.

If your overeating is accompanied by feeling very depressed, if you deliberately vomit or use laxatives to help you manage your feelings about eating or your size and shape, or if you hurt yourself in other ways, you may need to seek professional help rather than use this book on its own. It is also important to note that if you are significantly underweight – if your body mass index (BMI) is under 18 (see page 39 for how to work this out) – then you should seek medical support, either through your GP or from a professionally trained therapist. You can use some of the websites in the 'Useful resources' section to help you find advice.

As you work through this book, you will discover various examples of the complex relationship we can have with food. We will explore how a compassionate mind approach can help you to understand this, to move towards a non-dieting life, and gradually to accept yourself for who you are, including your size and shape. Moreover, it will help you find a place of fulfilment and happiness, and cope with life's inevitable ups and downs.

My personal reflections on Chapter 1

Please give yourself some time to think about the following key questions. You may like to write the answers down or to talk about them with someone else.

- What are your personal take-home messages from this chapter?

- How do you think developing a compassionate approach to eating and your body would help you?

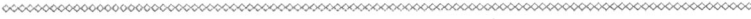

∞∞∞

SUMMARY

A compassionate approach always starts with understanding what we are up against.

- Our brains have not really evolved mechanisms for self-restraint; they did not need to because our eating was constrained by the relative shortage of food and our foraging survival style.

- Eating evolved to be a highly social event, is associated with soothing and can be used as a reward, but we can also use it to punish ourselves.

- Our problems with food can relate to complicated emotional difficulties.

- Modern Western societies have a damaging tendency to blame us for the problems that are the side effects of our new ways of living, and to see them as our individual, rather than collective, responsibility to sort out.

- Many of us take the blame for problems that are not our fault, resulting in us feeling inadequate, ashamed, helpless and hopeless in managing our eating and weight.

- Your struggle with food is absolutely *not your fault*.

This book will help you to compassionately understand your eating and emotions and learn to care for yourself without the need for dieting or overeating.

2 Making sense of over-eating, part 1 – how our bodies work

When survival skills backfire

As we saw in Chapter 1, our 'see-food-and-eat-it' brain gave us a massive evolutionary advantage in times of unpredictability, shortage or famine. So, we have a body that is very good at storing energy (as fat, muscle and glycogen) and able to survive for weeks at a time with a poor food supply. Indeed, it can even boost its immune system during periods of famine by absorbing essential minerals from our bones. Our body helps us survive by slowing down our reproductive system and the rate at which we burn energy. It even helps us manage the distress caused by being hungry; with a 'high' and extra burst of energy that stops us sleeping until we find the next available food source. People who diet can become somewhat addicted to this natural 'high'.

These remarkable survival skills first became potentially problematic when we moved from nomadic hunter-gatherer groups into agricultural economies. It then became a little easier to obtain a more regular supply of protein (from the meat of domestic animals or products from them such as milk, eggs or cheese).

The problems that we face now with eating habits and obesity only really emerged over the past two hundred years as we became more efficient at producing reliable and sustainable supplies of energy-dense and good-tasting food. We have moved away from the diet we evolved to eat (primarily fruit and vegetables, with a small amount of protein from fish and meat) to one of highly processed protein and carbohydrate, with only a relatively small proportion of fruit and vegetables; and at the same time we have significantly reduced the energy we use in day-to-day life.

We also evolved with a sweet tooth and a strong disgust response to food that might be contaminated or poisonous. Experiments clearly show that when good-tasting foods are available we tend to prefer them over bland foods – and we tend to eat more of them than we actually need. One of the consequences of eating sweet or sugary food is that it forces our body to increase production of a hormone called insulin, which is designed to 'sweep up' excess glucose in the blood. Once the extra insulin has gone to work, our 'blood sugar level' drops, and our body interprets this as us being hungry. The longer this cycle goes on, the more likely we are to want to eat more than we need, and the more likely it is that this will be stored as fat. This chapter and the next are designed to provide you with the information you need to begin to manage your body and brain, and in particular the complex relationship between your emotions, body shape, weight and eating.

Body issues

Although we share an evolutionary history, it is pretty obvious that we are not all the same. There are lots of ways in which we differ – for example, in height, hair colour, sporting talent and intellectual abilities. It is important to recognise that our bodies are not all the same when it comes to eating and weight gain, either. There are several important differences that we need to take into account when we consider these issues.

The ease with which we put on weight is linked to basic physiology. For example, there are cells in your body called 'brown fat cells', which regulate how much fat you lay down. Some ethnic groups tend to put on weight faster than others because their bodies are better adapted to survive in environments where food is scarce. We all know people who seem to be able to eat loads but do not put on weight. Some of them will have a faster metabolic rate, so they tend to burn the food they consume more quickly than others; some are more active – even when resting, they fidget more! – which both increases their metabolic rate and means they are using up more energy than people who are less active.

How easily we are satisfied by food also seems to vary. Some people, even when they are physically full, don't seem to experience the feeling of fullness. Many of us still feel able to put in a little bit more, having just an extra biscuit or bit of cheese. But for some it's more serious: they are constantly hungry. The scientific reasons for this are still being investigated and there remains much to learn about hunger, appetite and craving regulation.

As we've already seen, regulating our eating isn't just a matter of willpower, as many diet gurus try to tell us – but, yes, there are some people who seem to find it easier to control their desires than others. Why this should be so is also still a matter of scientific debate. We do know, however, that there are many things that can undermine willpower – for example, a lack of opportunities to learn to cope with our feelings, or unhelpful rules about how and what we are 'allowed' to eat. Psychological studies suggest that we can learn to develop willpower by creating helpful conditions for our efforts.

It's important to note, then, that the differences between us in terms of appetite and weight gain, our ability to recognise when we're full and even our willpower are in large part biologically determined, and therefore out of our hands. We may be able to learn to manage them differently, but we are not responsible for how and why they occurred in the first place.

Different cultures find different body shapes and sizes attractive. There are cultures where men and women seek to put on weight because plumpness signals possession of resources and status. Sumo wrestlers try desperately to put on weight because this is culturally attractive and gives them an advantage in the wrestling ring. There is nothing intrinsically attractive or unattractive in being large. However, in most Western cultures slimness and a high hip-to-waist ratio is now the culturally desired shape for women, and a flat stomach and well-defined muscles are the desired shape for men, with these body shapes indicating youth, health and success.

We live in a society that has become highly focused on how people look – which includes facial appearance, body size and clothes. A drive for a slim and young-looking body shape is partly linked to social and cultural definitions of what is attractive – and these in turn both feed off and are fed by consumer industries whose business is selling things.

If we cannot meet these goals, we often feel inferior and ashamed, and fearful of being rejected; so, we push ourselves to change our eating habits and our bodies to get closer to what we think is the 'ideal'. And when – as is so often the case – we can't reach our unrealistic goals, we can also become very self-critical.

Health issues

More pressure to eat and weigh less has come from an entirely different source. Medical science has recently shown that there is a link between weight and health. People with a body mass index (BMI) above a certain level are more likely to suffer from significant difficulties with blood pressure, vulnerability to diabetes, pressure on joints and so forth. Indeed, some of the health problems associated with being excessively overweight can be tragic. On the face of it, it's hard to argue with the message that we should avoid being overweight if it's doing us physical harm. But part of the problem with this message is that it comes with an associated idea that healthy is morally good and unhealthy is morally bad. This rather accusatory approach is reflected in the number of television programmes about losing weight where overweight people are targeted. In some cases, too, there are class undertones, with barely disguised suggestions that working-class people have poor diets because they are somehow lazy or can't be bothered to eat 'properly'. Again, all too often, concerns about the consequences of being overweight, whether based on medical or commercial motives, have come to be increasingly associated with shame and problems of self-control.

Increasingly, a healthy lifestyle is seen as a matter of choice, and failure to adopt one as shameful and weak. Indeed, some in the medical profession have even debated whether treatment should be withheld because resources are scarce and should not be 'squandered' on people who don't 'look after themselves'. Many of my clients have stories to tell about health professionals who have not been very sympathetic to their struggle. And yet there is plenty of evidence that it is really difficult to lose weight and keep it off in the long term, and that you don't need to lose very much weight to become healthy.

It is hard not to feel as if you are caught between two worlds – one that tells you cakes are 'naughty but nice' and hires popular football stars to advertise crisps, and one populated by people in white coats who imply there is something morally suspect about you if you can't control your weight. No wonder so many people struggle, and criticise themselves when they cannot exert perfect control over their appetite or desire for food!

It's also important to keep in mind that most of us rarely use our bodies for the things they evolved to do, namely the various kinds of physical activity that filled up the vast majority of most people's lives from hunter-gatherer times to the Middle Ages. Our working life has become more sedentary, and manual work has become the exception rather than the norm. We are far more likely to travel by car or public transport than by foot or bicycle, as our homes are further from our jobs; and fear of harm has meant that our children are less likely to walk to school, play outside, or even take part in some sports, while curriculum pressures have all too often resulted in less and less time being given to formal and informal physical activity in the school week. There is now real concern about the lack of physical activity that both we and our children undertake, but it's only recently that our governments have woken up to the problem and tried to introduce schemes to encourage us to be more active. Even if we want to be physically active, it can be difficult to fit exercise around our working and family lives. Cultural changes and constraints are no more our fault than is our biological make-up, and yet they do pose significant problems in how we manage our bodies.

I'm not suggesting for a moment that we should ignore these health issues or brush them under the carpet. It is the blaming and shaming that are wrong – because these just make us feel bad, and do not encourage or inspire us to try harder if we need to. An accusatory approach does not offer solutions and often makes it even less likely we will lose weight for the sake of our health.

My personal reflections on dieting

In this section, I invite you to pause your reading and think about your personal history with dieting. If you have felt pressure to lose weight (as many of us have), the following questions are designed to help you understand your relationship with weight loss and dieting. If this has been difficult for you, you are not alone; most people who diet find it difficult, but blame *themselves* for the diet not working, or motivate themselves though shame, fear and self-criticism. Very rarely do people sustain weight loss in the longer term, and many people end up yo-yo dieting. Again, you may wish to use these as discussion points with someone who cares about you, or as private written exercises:

- How many times in your life have you tried to lose weight?

- What did you hope losing weight would bring you (e.g. happiness, confidence, health benefits, etc.)?

- What pressures do you think led to you thinking that you needed to lose weight in the past?

- Are there any current pressures for you to lose weight?

- What has it been like trying to diet?

- How long could you keep your diet going?

- How have you motivated yourself to diet?

- How did you deal with the inevitable urges to eat when you dieted (e.g. trying harder, beating yourself up, giving up, etc.)?

- Can you imagine what life would be like if you stopped dieting? What would be your biggest fears of giving up dieting?

The answers to these questions will help you decide whether you want to carry on dieting, and therefore be prone to overeating, for the rest of your life, or if you want to try a new approach that helps to meet your emotional and physical needs without food being a major way of doing this.

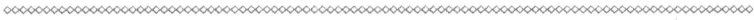

Aoife's story

We can get more insight into how complex these difficulties can be, and how mixed messages can make us feel ashamed and self-critical, by looking at one individual's experience. Aoife's story is typical of many people who have attempted to diet. It shows how something as supposedly easy as losing weight can be a very complicated and tricky business, and how this struggle can often be linked with other feelings we have about ourselves.

Aoife was in the 'healthy' weight range for her height, although her weight had fluctuated and at times in her life she had weighed much more. Whatever her weight, she always felt very dissatisfied with her body. While she was growing up, she was a little overweight for her height and was often teased by her peers about her appearance. She learned to think about her body all the time, because that was the aspect of her that attracted criticism, and also to be fearful of what people thought about her. She believed that the only way she could be accepted by others was to be thinner; and so, ever since her early teens, she has been on and off diets.

In some ways, Aoife was a relatively successful dieter. Although her weight fluctuated, she was able to keep it within the healthy weight range. However, she believed she needed to be constantly vigilant about what and when she ate. She had lots of rules about this and did her best to avoid eating socially so that people could not pressure her into eating things she thought she should not eat.

Like many dieters, Aoife often found that she could not keep to her strict rules for more than two or three months. When she gained weight after a diet (as most dieters will) she became very afraid, and after a week or two she would try to diet again. Aoife felt that the best way to keep her desire for her 'forbidden foods' and her hunger in check was to constantly call herself names – names like 'fatty', 'pig' and 'fat cow' – some of which she had learned from the children who had bullied and teased her when she was young, and others she had made up herself. Not surprisingly, Aoife felt low and miserable when she called herself these names. Because Aoife was fearful of her weight, and because it was associated in her mind with social unacceptability and shame, when she felt overweight those feelings of being pointed at and ashamed would return. This would then trigger a sinking feeling and a sense of frustration, which quickly turned into self-criticism: 'What's the matter with me? Why can't I keep to my diets?' Out of this would come feelings of anger and contempt, and more name-calling.

Sometimes, when she felt low, Aoife would stand in front of the mirror looking at bits of her body that she particularly didn't like and calling herself even more names. At other times she would scream and shout at herself as she tried on clothes (usually the ones she could only fit in at her lowest weight) or look at pictures of herself in the past and predict future misery if she did not lose weight. Sometimes Aoife could not stand the misery that dieting caused her and would have what she called a 'stuff it' moment, when she would give up dieting and eat a lot of her 'forbidden' foods. At these times, food would sometimes give her comfort and relief but also was a way of punishing herself.

Aoife's rejection of dieting showed a more rebellious side of her that was struggling to feel free – and in some ways was vital to her moving forward. However, as you can imagine, she had a real battle going on inside herself, between the angry, 'stuff it' part of her and the fear-driven part that wanted to control her eating. If we are honest, we can all feel that battle sometimes.

So, Aoife had two problems. One was linked to her eating and weight, and the other, more serious, was about her relationship with herself – which was negative, attacking and rejecting. Self-criticism of this type never creates confidence, encouragement, enthusiasm, sustained effort or genuine attempts to take responsibility. At best it can create a temporary, fearful falling-into-line, which is what it did for Aoife.

It is clear that her relationship with food and eating had little to do with managing her physical health. Rather, it was tied up with managing her painful memories, and her fear of bullying and rejection. Given how horrible these events made her school years, it is understandable that Aoife would try to manage her size and shape to avoid further rejection as an adult. But one of the unintended consequences of doing so was that she became a bully to herself, and she got caught up in a vicious circle of dieting, self-attack, low mood and binge-eating. This in turn left her feeling even more fearful of rejection by other people and led to her weight yo-yoing by about 13 kg, even though she remained in a 'healthy' weight range.

It is for people like Aoife that this book is written. Aoife was able to use many of the skills we will explore later to help her end this vicious cycle and develop a more compassionate relationship with her eating and her body.

My personal reflections on Aoife's story

You may wish to pause your reading again and spend some time reflecting on your experience of Aoife's story: how it connects (or doesn't) with your own, and whether it encourages you to explore a compassionate approach to understanding your relationship with eating.

- What did it feel like to read Aoife's story?

- Was there a part of you that was angry? If so, what made you feel this way?

- Was there a part of you that was sad? If so, what made you feel this way?

- Was there a part of you that was angry? If so, what made you feel this way?

- Was there a part of you that was critical of Aoife? If so, what made you feel this way?

- Is there a part of you that wants to find a compassionate way for Aoife (and other people) to manage their complex relationship with food and eating? If so, you may wish to continue reading this book and try out some of the exercises for yourself.

Food, eating and the need for self-compassion

Many of us live in a culture that dictates what our body size should be, and links this with success in our relationships and professional lives, and with our self-esteem. And yet I have never met anyone, in either my professional or my personal life (and that includes me), who is completely happy with their body size and shape. Indeed, all of us can find fault with parts of our bodies if we look hard enough. If you don't believe this, imagine standing right in front of a mirror and looking closely at a part of your body you feel happy with, trying to spot small flaws and imperfections. If you tell yourself that these things are important and will have a bearing on how other people see you or treat you, you will find an easy path to dissatisfaction with your body. In fact, when people are anxious about their looks, that's exactly what they sometimes do – stare into the mirror looking for flaws. When we focus in like this, our brain can easily give us a feeling of dissatisfaction, even with things we were satisfied with before!

On the other hand, we know that the numbers of people who are very overweight – that is, clinically obese, which is defined as having a BMI of 35 or over, or morbidly obese (having a BMI over 40) – are rising sharply. Recent estimates suggest that more than 25 per cent of adults in the UK are now clinically obese; this is almost double the rate of ten years ago. In the USA, 31 per cent of adults are estimated to have a BMI over 30. And the picture is even worse for our children, whose overall levels of obesity and rates of increase are higher than those of their parents.

As we have already seen, there is a range of reasons why obesity has become such a serious problem. It's very clear that the cause of the problem lies not in individuals but in our societies.

You might think, then, that it would best be tackled by trying to develop social interventions that target the food industry and increase activity levels. In fact, quite the opposite has happened, with yet another industry flourishing – the diet industry.

Most diets tell us that significant reductions in energy intake and increases in energy output through exercise will give us complete control over our size and shape. There is also the suggestion that weight loss is both desirable and sustainable for everyone. Anyone who has been on a diet, or seen their friends and family dieting, will probably know that things are not this straightforward. Indeed, the evidence suggests that most diets, and particularly those involving severe or rapid weight loss, are likely to end in failure, and in all probability further weight gain. Furthermore, dieting can have significant physical and psychological consequences, particularly if your weight goes up and down repeatedly – known as 'yo-yo dieting' – or you lose it too rapidly. There is also the psychological harm that can arise if we keep trying and failing at things, which doesn't exactly inspire confidence or build self-esteem – and yet this is the common experience of dieters.

We need to recognise that it's important that we eat enough healthy food, maintain a relatively stable and healthy body weight, and provide our body with the degree of both physical activity and rest that it needs. We also need to take responsibility, as best we can, for doing all these things, despite living in a society that doesn't really help us. So we have to find a way of helping ourselves; and, as we will see in the rest of this book, that means learning to be deeply compassionate in tackling these difficulties so that we can feel encouraged and supported, are able to 'fail' without feeling ashamed or critical, and can just pick ourselves up and keep going.

What is a 'healthy body weight'?

Let's now look more deeply into the health aspects of weight. Medical professionals today calculate a 'healthy body weight' using something called the body mass index, or BMI, which I've already referred to. It's not hard to work out your own BMI. First, multiply your height in metres by itself. Then divide your weight in kilograms by this number. The number you end up with is your BMI. (You might want to look at www.nhs.uk/health-assessment-tools/calculate-your-body-mass-index to help you calculate your BMI.)

For example, Aoife weighs 70 kilograms (11 stone) and is 1.7 metres (5 feet 7 inches) tall. So, to work out her BMI she would first multiply 1.7 by 1.7, giving a figure of 2.89, and then divide 70 by 2.89. This gives her BMI, which is just over 24. People with a BMI in the range 20–25 are believed to have a healthy body weight. So, Aoife could weigh anything between 58 kg (9 st 2 lb) and 75 kg (11 st 10 lb) – a range of 17 kg, or 2 st 6 lb – and still be at a healthy weight for her height. This gives people considerable scope in what their healthy weight can be and represents a move away from the old-fashioned (and unsustainable) very narrow 'ideal weight' bands, which were mainly based upon the dictates of fashion rather than health.

Many health professionals believe that risks to our health increase significantly if we have a BMI of over 30 or below 18. However, even this wider band – at the upper end, at least – has been questioned. There is now good evidence to suggest that some people with a BMI of over 30 may face significantly fewer health risks than people who are in the 'healthy' weight range, if they are physically active and eat healthily according to their body's needs.

There are many myths around healthy body weight. As we've already seen, obesity is on the rise in many Western countries, and very substantial excess weight – described by medical professionals as 'morbid obesity' – does pose risks to health. However, there are other statistics to be taken into account. We are collectively a bit heavier (around 2.7 kg to 5.9 kg) than the previous generation, but we are also taller (2.5 cm on average) and are likely to live up to seven years longer.

So, there's no need to panic. The key issue is not to let collective changes blind us to our own individual needs, or automatically to assume that we need to lose weight. We may live in a culture where being a little taller and heavier than our parents is actually more likely to mean we are healthy – if we also eat what our body needs and are physically active. However, if we overeat a lot – especially if we eat a lot of foods that are not particularly good for us – and are much heavier than we would be if we ate what our body needed, then it can only be a good thing to address this in a compassionate manner.

So, we know, then, that our bodies can be healthy in a relatively wide weight range. When we are at a healthy body weight, we can function to the best of our abilities, physically, intellectually and emotionally. It's important to realise that it's often not weight itself that poses risks to our health so much as not caring for our bodies by providing them with consistent levels of adequate nutrition and activity. Attempts to achieve rapid weight loss are no more likely to improve our health than rapid or prolonged weight gain. Weight does play a role in our health, but as one of a wide range of other factors.

How our bodies regulate their own weight: the set point system

Our bodies have evolved to maintain a set weight, which is determined by factors such as genetics and the level of nutrition received in the womb or as a child. People who do not diet or overeat very much tend to maintain a relatively stable weight throughout their adult lives. When weight changes do occur, biological mechanisms (e.g. increases/decreases in appetite, changes in body metabolism) then act to restore weight to a stable level. A model known as 'set point theory' has been developed to help us understand this. The 'set point' evolved to maintain our body weight at a level that is healthy for each of us. It is possible to override it, but it takes a great deal of effort to keep our weight below our set point in the long term, and doing so poses a significant risk to our health. Our bodies find it easier to maintain our weight above our set point, but again this can also affect our health.

In animals and young children, the set point is relatively easily maintained by the hunger–satiety system – in plain English, whether we feel empty or full. As we grow up, our relationship with food becomes far more complex and we can choose to ignore this system – for example, by not eating when we are hungry or eating when we feel full. Our bodies are able to cope with day-to-day fluctuations (for example, overdoing it at Christmas) and will normally restore our body weight by short-term changes in our appetite and metabolic rate. However, our bodies have not evolved to cope with prolonged periods of starvation, overeating or irregular eating patterns. These can override our body's natural ability to stabilise our weight. Our bodies also work on a 'better safe than sorry' principle, which evolved in times when famine was a constant threat. So, if we do lose a significant amount of weight and then go back to eating normally again, our set point goes up to allow us to gain more weight in defence against future 'famine'. This is why, on average, a person who goes on a diet ends up in the long term 1.3 kg heavier than they were before they began.

The set point system is a complex one. Our body regulates our weight and eating through two main mechanisms: the rate at which our body naturally uses up energy (the metabolic rate), and our experiences of feeling hungry or having had enough food (the hunger–satiety system). In addition, there are several ways in which the natural 'set point' mechanism can be overridden: some of them involve deliberate attempts to manage our weight or feelings, while others happen without any direct intention on our part. These are shown in Figure 2.1.

Figure 2.1 Ways we can override the hunger–satiety system

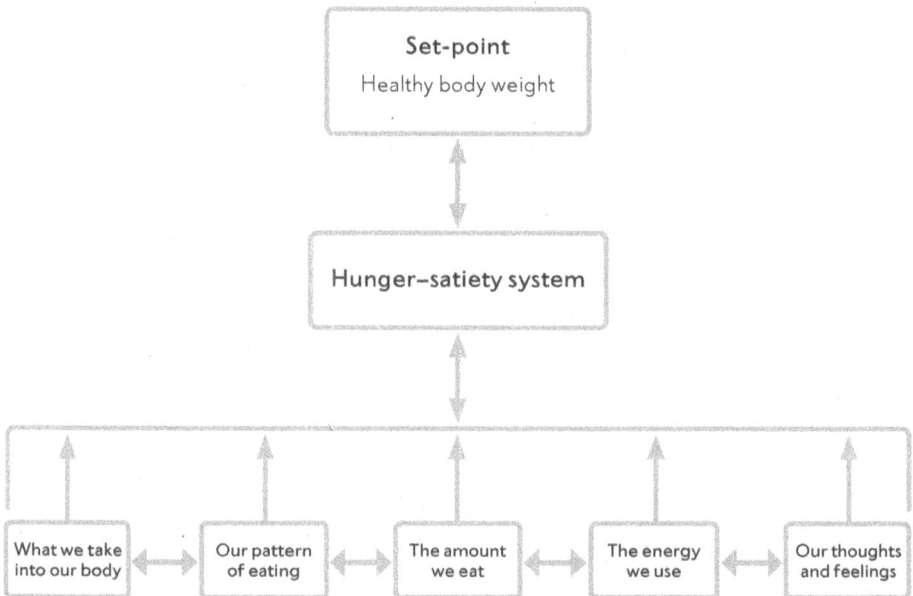

Overeating, set point and the hunger-satiety system

In the remainder of this chapter, we will explore how changing our set point can happen via the body's natural response to things we take into it, our eating patterns, and the amount of energy we eat and use up (the first four boxes in the bottom row of Figure 2.1). In Chapter 3, we will explore the complex relationship between our social relationships, emotions and eating (the last box in the bottom row of the figure). We will see how central self-criticism is to many people's attempts to manage their eating – even, in some cases, turning into self-disgust and self-loathing.

As a result of (probably unwittingly) altering the balance of your hunger–satiety system, it's quite probable that you will be out of touch with, or afraid of, your body's natural response to hunger or to being overfed. This section is designed to help you understand this system and to begin to work with it, rather than against it, as you develop a healthier relationship with eating.

What we take into our bodies
Fluid

Besides air, food is the third most important thing that we take into our body – the second most important is, of course, fluid. How much we drink can have a significant effect on our eating and our health. Many weight loss diets advise people to drink a glass or more of water before or during eating so they will feel full and hence eat less.

Given its importance, it is not surprising that we have evolved powerful and complex mechanisms for dealing with fluid intake, just as we have for hunger. If we eat less, we also tend to drink less, and the more we eat, the more we need to drink. Training our bodies to drink water rather than eat when we are hungry can upset this mechanism and will leave us feeling full, even bloated. It can also make it very difficult for us to know when we have had too much (or too little) food. If we drink far too much, particularly without eating, this can lead to imbalances in the body that can seriously affect our health, and in the most extreme cases kill us.

Over 70 per cent of our weight is made up of fluid. Rapid weight loss is often seen as desirable in diet programmes, but this usually relies on dehydration and so is not sustainable in the long term – as soon as we put fluid back into our body, the weight tends to go back on and even increase for a while. What happens when we lose weight rapidly, through dieting or a lot of activity, is that we lose water and glycogen. Glycogen is starch, and we store 0.5–1.5 kg of it in our liver and muscles. It is the body's equivalent of rocket fuel, an easily accessible source of energy. Understandably, the body does not like running out of this handy resource, and if it runs low, we snatch it back as soon as some carbohydrate is eaten. Glycogen needs to be stored in solution, and we need 0.5–1.3 litres of water to store 0.5 kg of glycogen. So, if you use up 0.5 kg of glycogen you will actually lose 1–2 kg total weight. Conversely, if you put back 0.5 kg of glycogen, you will gain 1–2 kg total weight.

Suppose that you go on a strict diet for a week before your holiday, eating very little and going to the gym and for a run every day. By the end of the week the scales tell you that you've lost 3.5 kg. You're delighted – now you can feel better on the beach. On holiday you eat normally – not excessively – and do a fair bit of walking and swimming, but nothing very energetic. You get home and stand on the scales and are horrified to discover that not only have you put that 3.5 kg back on but you've also put on another 1 kg! All that has happened is that you lost 1 kg of glycogen in that week of near starvation, which took another 2.5 kg of water with it. This sudden depletion of your glycogen stores rang warning bells in your body, so as soon as you started eating some carbohydrates again it made sure to get back all the glycogen it could, replacing more than the amount you lost so that, with the extra water needed to store it, you gained a little more weight than you'd lost in the first place. Not very encouraging, is it?

Alcohol and other drugs

It's all too easy to think that weight is all about food, and in fact we are often unaware of the effects that other things we put in our bodies can have on our eating and weight. It is not surprising, given the prejudice and stigma attached to being even a little overweight, that some people are so desperate to change that they will deliberately take legal and illegal drugs in their attempts to lose weight. These include:

- laxatives
- diuretics (e.g. caffeine)
- amphetamines
- diet pills
- thyroxin
- insulin (necessary for diabetics, but sometimes misused)
- cigarettes.

It is important to acknowledge that these do work, at least in the short term, for some people. Some of these drugs (such as diet pills) will affect appetite directly; others (such as cigarettes) are likely to be used as a substitute for food or for emotional eating. All carry health risks – for example, smoking is linked to cancer, and caffeine to disturbed sleep – and most people are likely to gain weight when they stop using them. Some, such as diuretics and laxatives, give the illusion of weight loss, but, as we have seen, this is usually by causing rapid fluctuations in fluid content that are not translated into long-term weight loss.

So, while taking any of these drugs can often give a sense of control over weight gain, it is likely that this will be at best short-lived. It may actually make things worse, as we give ourselves permission to overeat because we will later be taking something to get rid of the food (such as a laxative).

Other people may deliberately or accidentally stimulate their hunger by taking:

- alcohol

- antihistamines

- steroids

- some antidepressants or anti-psychotic medication

- marijuana.

These are substances that people often take to manage difficult feelings, without recognising the longer-term effects they are likely to have on our mood, appetite or ability to manage our eating. Some people, of course, have no choice but to take medication to manage medical or psychiatric conditions; however, they are often not aware of the side effects this will have for their weight.

Perhaps the most interesting, and certainly the most widely used, of these substances is alcohol. Most of us know it contains a lot of calories and reduces our inhibitions – including those about eating. More importantly, it also stimulates appetite in the short term (how else could I explain the desperate need for a kebab at 2 a.m.?). Although in the short-term alcohol can feel as if it relaxes us and helps us feel good, it can actually have a negative effect on our mood, leaving us wanting another drink when we come home at the end of the hectic evening. That extra glass of wine reduces our inhibitions more, which in turn reduces our ability to eat sensibly – and we raid the fridge for snacks. Then in the morning we feel annoyed with ourselves again. This is a very common cycle – and most of us never stop to ask ourselves if maybe the lifestyles we're leading, that send us to alcohol for relaxation, are just too stressful. So, the role it plays in our weight is complex. It is linked to the amount we drink and its effect on our moods, our appetites and our ability to resist our desires.

Our pattern of eating

Our eating patterns can have a profound effect on our body's natural mechanism for regulating our weight. We live in a world that makes extreme and conflicting demands on us. Often it is difficult to respond to our natural urges to eat regularly, for example because we work in jobs that do not allow us time to take proper breaks to look after our bodies, or because we are running around looking after a house and children and rarely have time for a proper meal. On the other hand, our culture promotes the belief that exercising extreme control over our eating habits is the only way to manage our weight – or even to be happy!

There are three major eating patterns that people who overeat tend to fall into:

1.   the starve–eat cycle

2.   the starve–binge–purge cycle

3.   chaotic eating.

The starve–eat cycle

Many people will at some time deliberately attempt to lose weight, either by restricting eating or exercising more, or both. As a result 'biological starvation' takes place; this is when our body is using up more energy than it is consuming. The body's natural response is to make us want to eat. This was the pattern we evolved to help us deal with times of famine, to encourage us to go looking for more food.

We learned a lot about what happens to the human body when it is deprived of adequate nutrition in the late 1940s and 1950s, when psychologists and doctors tried to work out how to safely re-feed famine and concentration camp victims after the end of the Second World War. A pioneering study found that even at the calorie levels suggested by most diet programmes, volunteers experienced profound psychological and physical side effects. These included:

- preoccupation with food and eating

- episodes of overeating

- low mood and irritability

- becoming obsessional

- difficulty in concentrating

- loss of interest in everyday activities

- loss of sexual desire

- feeling unsociable

- relationship difficulties.

The starvation response appears to follow a specific pattern with two distinct phases: initially the body drives us to find food, and then, if these attempts fail, it helps us to conserve energy stores. The side effects of these responses can reinforce our attempts to lose weight, particularly in the early stages of a diet. However, the effects in phase two can often lead to weight gain, and in turn to fear of our appetite and desire for food. It's worth going into a bit of detail here about how the starvation response works in someone who goes on a diet, if we are to understand why attempts to manage our weight so often founder.

Phase 1: The initial search for food

Weight loss is relatively easy in the early weeks of dieting, mainly because we lose fluid and glycogen first. This can help motivate us further to continue with our diet.

In these first weeks we get an initial burst of energy and tend to feel in a good mood (a 'starvation high'). This response evolved to help us get up and look for food. So, if we are dieting, we learn (at least in the early stages) that eating less makes us feel better. We learn to associate not eating with feeling good.

So far, so good. But the next feature of this phase often causes problems. Food becomes more important than anything else. We become preoccupied with thoughts of food and eating, and more sensitised to food smells or taste. So, we will often be more tempted by foods than usual. If we 'give in' and eat them, we often (wrongly) see this as a lack of willpower and can become very self-critical of our 'weakness'.

Another effect is that we become more emotionally detached – that is, our feelings become somewhat blunted – because when we were really starving, we could not afford to let any emotional distractions get in the way of our search for food and survival. Again, if we're dieting it seems to us that losing weight actually does help us manage our emotions.

We also find it more difficult to sleep and may become more restless, because we cannot afford to rest when we need to look for food to survive. Problems with sleep are common in people who diet, and sleep deprivation in turn has a profound effect on our appetite. When we are tired, we tend to produce more of the hormones that make us feel hungry: we feel less full, and our appetite increases. We also become depressed and irritable. None of this is good news for those of us who are anxious about eating more, or who tend to eat to manage our feelings.

As we lose weight our body adjusts our metabolic rate downwards to conserve energy, so it becomes harder to lose more weight (what dieters call a 'plateau'). This is very frustrating; it often drives us to even more extreme attempts at weight loss or into the starve–binge–purge pattern we will look at next.

Phase 2: Losing the hunt for food

As we lose more weight and cannot find food, the body starts to take emergency steps to preserve energy:

- It stops pumping blood to our fingers and toes, to reduce heat loss.

- It slows down the rate at which we empty our stomach, leading to problems of constipation and bloating (so we feel very full).

- We are even less able to concentrate.

- We feel exhausted. By this point our rate of weight loss has slowed down even more: we have given up the hunt for food and our only hope is to stop moving and survive until someone brings it to us.

- We experience mood swings, feeling increasingly detached from everyday living, and tend to isolate ourselves from others. This may be an evolved response to save us from the distress of our imminent death and allow our families to leave us and carry on the hunt for food.

- Eventually our body begins to eat itself to survive, it gets vitamins and minerals from our bones (giving us osteoporosis), and starts to draw on our vital organs and muscles to provide calories.

- Finally, if there is still no food coming in, we die.

Of course, most of us who diet will not get to the last stage of this sequence! But there is good evidence to suggest that those who lose weight by deliberately giving the body less than it needs for long periods of time will experience problems with their physical and psychological health. Fortunately, as we will see in later chapters, managing your weight doesn't have to be a constant battle with your own survival instincts: the body has very good ways of judging how much it needs to eat, and if we trust it and learn to listen to it, our health will benefit as a result.

The eating response to starvation

Just as our bodies have evolved a fixed set of responses to the absence of food, so they have also evolved very efficient survival mechanisms to make the most of food when it becomes available again. These affect:

- what food we eat

- how fast we eat

- how our weight changes.

Our initial response to starvation is to try to eat – anything! This includes things we would not normally contemplate. At the most extreme, this can mean eating things that are otherwise taboo for religious or cultural reasons (including animals or even other humans). In less extreme circumstances, it can mean eating things we really don't like: how many of us have found ourselves, late at night in the kitchen, hoovering up unappetising leftovers or eating cold baked beans from the tin? Yes, I thought it wasn't just me!

As most dieters have a lot of rules in place about what they can and can't eat, this drive can cause real difficulties. We can become very self-critical when we break our rules, seeing ourselves as weak or inadequate in some way when all we're doing is responding to our body's natural need to recover from a famine – even if it's one we have imposed on ourselves.

Also, once food is available again, we usually eat more and faster than we would normally. In evolutionary terms this makes sense if we do not know where our next meal is coming from. For a dieter it seems that a week's 'success' can be wiped out in ten minutes.

As we have been eating less, our body has already slowed our metabolic rate down to conserve energy; this means that, when we start eating again, our weight tends to rise relatively rapidly, and at first it will stabilise at a higher weight than before the 'famine' began. This is the 'better safe than sorry' principle in action, giving us extra energy stores, particularly in the form of fat, in case famine returns. This can be very disappointing if we have deliberately tried to lose weight and it often sparks another spate of dieting. Many serial dieters will recognise this repeated cycle. In fact, if you want to gain weight the best way to do it is to diet!

Now for some more good news. Our body does not continually gain weight if food supplies are enough for our needs. Gradually our metabolic rate and eating return to normal, and as excess energy stores are no longer necessary, we gradually lose weight to our pre-diet level – but only if we don't diet again. However strange this may sound to habitual dieters, if the food supply continues to be adequate, and our activity levels don't exceed our need for food, then gradually eating and weight return to normal.

The starve–binge–purge cycle

When we go without food for more than three or four hours, it becomes increasingly difficult to ignore our body's drive to find and eat food in order to survive. After this time our blood sugar falls, and we produce hormones that stimulate our appetite. If we eat, particularly if we eat foods with some fat in them, this will turn off these hormones and trigger other hormonal changes that give us feelings of fullness, so we stop eating. We have already explored the various ways we can override this system, particularly by dieting. If we were in a genuine famine, our body's drive to find food would mean that when we came across any, we would eat as much as possible in order to replenish our energy supplies.

Eating larger amounts of food than is normal in an uncontrolled fashion is referred to as 'binge-eating' or 'bingeing'. However, whereas primitive men and women at the end of a famine would relax and tuck in, finding the presence of food a reason for rejoicing, people who are deliberately trying to lose weight or control their food intake tend to find bingeing a very upsetting experience. They often do not understand or are scared of their body's attempts to push them back to a healthy weight and an adequate intake of food. They tend to experience feelings of fear (of weight gain and of loss of control), guilt, shame and panic about wanting/needing to eat.

These feelings can then lead them to the 'purge' stage of the cycle, to get rid of the food they have eaten. Purging includes any method of getting rid of calories or food itself (e.g. excessive exercise, vomiting or use of laxatives). As well as having dangerous physiological effects, these reactions also make the body feel it is being starved even more. Most people who diet will recognise this cycle, even if only in a mild form that sends them off to the gym for an hour after eating half a packet of biscuits. In its most extreme form, it is the pattern associated with the eating disorder bulimia nervosa. However, most dieters are more likely to follow episodes of bingeing with further episodes of dieting. This pattern tends to lead to weight gain, mainly because of the effects of dieting on our metabolic rate that we looked at earlier.

So, you can see how this pattern can become a vicious circle of dieting, bingeing and purging, which is emotionally very difficult to manage and can have very serious health consequences. Figure 2.2 shows how this cycle fits together.

Figure 2.2 The starve–binge–purge cycle

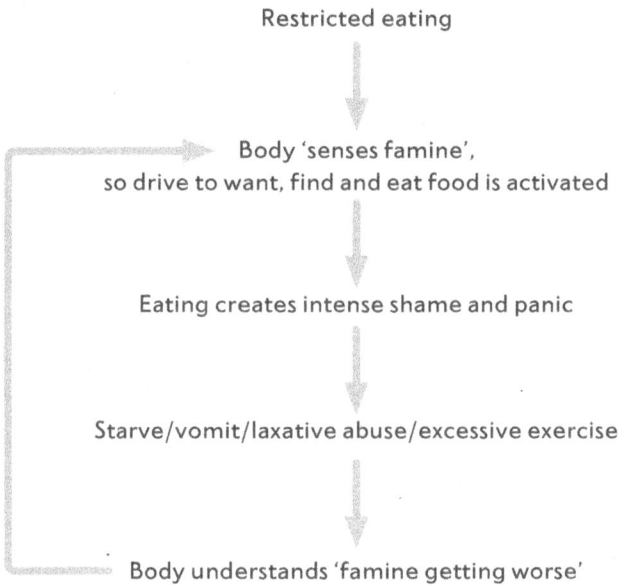

Restricted eating

↓

Body 'senses famine',
so drive to want, find and eat food is activated

↓

Eating creates intense shame and panic

↓

Starve/vomit/laxative abuse/excessive exercise

↓

Body understands 'famine getting worse'

Chaotic eating

Of course, most of us, when we are trying to do something about
our weight, do not fall neatly into mild versions of the starve–eat
or starve–binge–purge cycles. Some of us may fluctuate between
the two. Some find that even thinking about beginning a diet
can trigger an eating response. This may be particularly true for
'serial' dieters. Many of us find that our eating just becomes chaotic, veering between episodes of dieting and overeating, so that
we lose any sense of what it is to eat 'normally'. The important
thing for us to remember is that if we eat chaotically, our body
will tend to be on higher alert for signs of famine and so is likely
to trigger the hunger response more readily.

It is possible for our body to respond to our need to eat even if
we try to stop eating. For example, some people develop what
is called 'night eating disorder'. This is a form of sleepwalking

where individuals may not be aware of what they are eating because they do it while they are asleep. Others may develop a bingeing pattern but cannot or do not attempt to compensate by purging or restricting their food intake and so may put on weight. This weight gain leads to an increase in their metabolic rate. So, to maintain their weight at the new level they will initially feel hungrier than before or feel hungry even when they are full. This may mean they eat more in the long term, possibly leading to further gradual weight gain.

Some dieters can keep to their strict rules most of the time but, when they break them, have the 'stuff it' response. They get angry with themselves for breaking their diet and decide that if they have broken a rule they might as well break it properly! This can lead to binge-eating. Yet others may use food to punish themselves for being unable to keep to their diet.

These patterns are followed the world over by people who diet. Remember they are just a normal human response to trying to diet and lose weight. If you think about the number of rules when you are on a diet, you'll see that it is impossible to keep to them all – our natural need to eat means that you will break some. If you criticise yourself or see your desire to eat as a sign of personal weakness, this may motivate you to start dieting again, but it is also likely to lead to a lifetime struggling with your weight, eating and mood.

The amount we eat

The amount of food we eat can have a significant impact on how hungry or full we are, but as we are exploring in chapters 2 and 3, how much we eat is influenced by many things, not just whether we have eaten enough to manage our daily energy needs. Eating enough can help to reduce overeating. However, working out how much we need can be tricky and is reliant on many factors, including our body weight and the energy we use. Most of us are not good at estimating how much food we need, so we will explore this in more detail in Chapter 13 and help to get in touch with feelings of hunger and fullness in Chapter 15, to guide our eating in the long term.

The energy we use

Having looked at the intake side of the equation, let's now look at the output side. All the energy we get comes from food, and we use it in three ways:

1. to keep our body ticking over – for example, to keep our hearts beating, our blood going round and all our other vital organs functioning

2. to digest the food we eat

3. to fuel whatever activity we do.

If we eat just the amount of food we need for these three things, we are in 'energy balance'. That is, 'energy in' equals 'energy out': we do not store energy, nor are we deprived of it, and our weight remains stable. If we eat more energy than we use, it is stored as fat to be used at a later date. If we eat less energy than we use, our body interprets this as biological starvation and responds in the ways we saw in the previous section.

Ticking over

The largest portion of the energy we use up every day (between 60 and 75 per cent) is used just to keep our bodies functioning. The energy we eat is measured in calories, and most adults need about 1,400 calories per day just to 'tick over'. This would keep us alive if all we did was to lie completely still. The rate at which we use energy (without doing anything other than lying still) is called our 'resting metabolic rate' (RMR). Our RMR increases when we eat more, and decreases when we eat less than we need, as the body tries to conserve its dwindling energy stocks. There are also small differences between individuals in metabolic rates: for example, people with a higher proportion of muscle and bone, compared to fat, tend to have a higher metabolic rate, and it tends to reduce a little as we get older. But the requirement for about 1,400 calories a day is a pretty good rule of thumb.

Digestion

Eating and digesting food uses energy – but not much: on average, around 150 calories a day. So, to cover our RMR and the 'cost' in energy of taking in energy, we need to consume something like 1,550 calories a day.

Physical activity

Of course, none of us actually lies still all day, every day – so to calculate the total number of calories we use, we have to add those we need to maintain our RMR, those we use up eating and digesting, and those we need to fuel whatever physical activity we do. This includes all the ordinary things like walking to the bathroom and moving paper across the desk, as well as 'taking exercise' like playing football or going to the gym. Most women who are neither very inactive nor extremely active will use something between 2,000 and 2,500 calories per day. On average men tend to use more due to differences in body composition and will use around 2,500 to 3,000 calories per day.

This third area of energy use is the most variable. For example, someone who does no physical activity may need to add just 100 calories to the 1,550 they need for their body to tick over and to feed itself; whereas someone who is very active may need to add 3,000 calories a day to the same basic 1,550.

Interestingly, just as the body responds to our eating too little by slowing down energy use, if we eat too much it responds by trying to use up more. There is wide variation in how well our bodies do this, but everyone tends to increase their physical activity when they eat more. Scientists have proven what I call the 'Boxing Day effect' – the overwhelming desire to go for a walk after eating too much on Christmas Day! They found that humans naturally increase their physical activity after being forced to eat more than their body needs. Much of this appeared to be involuntary (i.e. fidgeting). If we tune in to this mechanism, even if we do overeat it is unlikely that we will gain weight.

Much of the information put out by the diet industry does not focus on the significant effects exercise can have on metabolic rate and health, implying that restricting eating, particularly by following low-calorie diets, will do the trick. In fact, as we have already seen, because our bodies have well-established health mechanisms, the most likely outcome is that our metabolic rate will slow down. On the other hand, even moderately increasing physical activity has a beneficial effect on both our physical and our psychological health. It works with our bodies by helping them to increase their metabolic rate, which in turn will help us to avoid gaining weight – as long as we put in enough calories to stop our body going into a starvation state.

Excessive exercise and activity

As I have just said, regular enjoyable exercise and activity can improve our physical and mental health. However, some people use exercise not only as a way of keeping fit and relaxed but as a way to try to reduce their weight below its natural set point, to alter their natural shape or to manage difficult feelings. I am not suggesting physical activity is a bad thing – far from it! However, it is important to recognise the potentially damaging effects that too much exercise can have on our health. For example:

- If no additional calories are taken in to compensate for those used in excessive exercise our body will read this sustained energy loss as 'famine', and this can trigger the starve–eat cycle or the starve–binge–purge cycle.

- Excessive exercise can do physical damage, for example to joints and muscles.

- If exercise becomes an obsession, this can do psychological damage: for example, we may start to get depressed, agitated, angry or anxious if we are unable to exercise as much as we want to.

- Obsessive exercise can also damage our social, personal and working lives if we get to the point of putting it ahead of other areas of life.

If you're not sure whether you might be exercising excessively, a good way to approach the question is to ask yourself if you treat your body like a professional athlete would treat theirs. They have planned rest days, will not exercise if they are ill or injured, maintain adequate levels of food intake, and tend to enjoy what their body can do for them.

My personal reflections on Chapter 2

Set point theory can be difficult to read about. It is common for people to have very mixed feelings about this, as popular culture is dominated by ideas about how easy it is to lose weight and how inadequate people are if they cannot simply follow a diet.

Our reaction to the notion of a set point can often help us reach a more compassionate understanding of why eating is difficult for ourselves and others. Accepting and learning to live with our set point can come with costs (e.g. sadness at the time spent dominated by dieting, concerns about how else you might accept and value your body without losing weight). Please spend some time thinking about your initial reactions to set point theory. These questions may be helpful to guide you:

- Have you ever been at a stable weight when you have not been dieting or overeating? If so, what was this like for you physically and emotionally?

- How have you tried to change your set point in the past?

- How long did it work for?

- Did it come with a cost to you in terms of your emotional, physical and social wellbeing?

- What are your biggest fears about discovering your personal set point by using this book?

- Can you imagine a world where you are not trying to change your body size and shape, either by dieting or deliberately/accidentally overeating?

- What would you need to be able to think and feel to let yourself do this?

SUMMARY

We humans have evolved a complex system to help us manage our eating in times of famine and make the most of food when the famine passes. This system is sensitive to a whole range of deliberate or accidental changes in our eating and appetite. Sometimes we can become afraid of, or even blame ourselves for, our body's natural attempts to stabilise our weight at a level that is healthy for us. Learning to take a compassion focused approach to this area of our lives will involve coming to understand more about the ways in which we have affected our 'set point' weight and getting back in touch with our body's natural systems for managing our weight and eating. Many people find this very difficult, particularly as it involves ignoring the advice that many give and the hope that it offers – that, if only we could keep to a low-calorie diet, we could all be as thin as we want, and that this is the path to happiness!

In the next chapter, we will explore how our feelings can influence our eating, and how we can learn different ways to deal with our difficult emotions.

3 Making sense of overeating, part 2 – eating and our feelings

In Chapter 2, we explored the ways in which we can deliberately or accidentally interfere with our body's natural ways of keeping us healthy and managing our urges to overeat. Perhaps the most powerful way in which we override these mechanisms is in response to factors in our social environment and to our emotional states.

Now, emotions are tricky things. Our basic emotions – our capacity to feel anger, anxiety, sadness, joy and lust – are older than our human species, having evolved many millions of years ago. They can be easily activated and can be powerful because they are accompanied by the surge through our bodies of chemicals called hormones. This means that when we feel strong emotions they arouse in us desires and urges to act – to fight, run away, cry or celebrate. Sometimes, if we have not learned to recognise, understand or cope with our emotions, they can seem overwhelming. Sometimes we can worry that if we don't control them, we will simply fall apart.

Also, of course, we can have a conflict of emotions. We can be very angry with somebody we love, so because we don't want to hurt them, we don't say anything but still feel resentful; or we can be very angry with somebody we're frightened of, so again we don't say anything, but later become angry and berate ourselves: 'Why don't I stand up for myself?'. We can be criticised for being too emotional or not emotional enough. Often our feelings (or at least showing them) can be seen as a sign of weakness, or a source of fear or shame. Interestingly, there seem to be different rules about feelings and how to handle them for different genders and cultures. These messages can be quite confusing: for example, 'men don't cry' (but 'new men' should), or 'women shouldn't show anger' (but 'new women' should).

Many people use food to deal with their emotions. Sometimes as children they were given food (chocolates, sweets, cakes) when they were upset. So instead of talking about thinking about their feelings they've learned simply to try to turn them off by distracting themselves with food. As they grow up, this becomes a way of life and allowing oneself to feel and think about one's emotions can seem very frightening. In this chapter, we will explore our emotions and how they can affect our eating.

Learning to eat

We will begin our journey by considering how feeding as an infant affects our emotions.

We know that suckling has a positive emotional impact. Infants show a typical pattern of being soothed and relaxed while feeding; but this also requires active involvement from the person doing the feeding. If baby mammals are given food, but not physical closeness, emotional warmth and eye contact, they become distressed when eating. They can even fail to grow and refuse to eat. So, from a very early stage we learn to associate food and eating with emotional comfort. Indeed, some psychologists have suggested that the feeding process actually provides the beginning of social and emotional development.

We have already seen that some of our food preferences are part of our biological make-up. However, we also learn a lot about the foods we like (or dislike), and when to stop eating them, as we grow up. For example, by two years of age toddlers know when they are full but also have learned from adults what foods are supposed to be eaten for breakfast. As we grow older, we learn to express certain food preferences and will even choose what foods we will eat in different situations. Most of us will remember some foods we would eat at school but never dream of eating at home. How we eat can also depend on what we learn from those around us. All too often these days meals are eaten on the go, so we have very little chance to recognise the tastes and textures of food, or the pleasure and feelings of fullness and satisfaction that taking time over eating can provide.

As we grow older, we become more aware of the social nature of eating, and how it can be used to celebrate or reward, as a distraction or to soothe emotional distress. We also learn that refusing food can be very upsetting for people around us. Eating (or refusing to eat) particular types of food can become part of our religious or moral identity.

Our eating changes as we move from childhood into adolescence. In these years we require far more energy to fuel the changes our body will make, and we also tend to become more physically active. These rapid growth spurts can leave us feeling very hungry a lot of the time: ask anyone with a teenager how often they need to refill the refrigerator! In our teens we tend to 'graze', snacking little and often. If we are left to grow through this normal stage, we will gradually learn to eat more regularly again and are unlikely to overeat in the long run. Yet there are many social pressures, particularly on teenagers, to moderate or even limit their eating, and so many start forcing their eating into restrictive patterns, or into patterns that are fine for younger children and adults (who need less food) – for example, leaving longer gaps between meals, perhaps eating breakfast and having only a small lunch – and are discouraged from snacking. As a consequence, they are actually more likely to end up overeating.

This period of growth is particularly important when we are trying to understand the link between our emotions and eating. As children faced with the physical changes that come just before and during puberty, we naturally become preoccupied with the size and shape of ourselves and other people. We are also learning to deal with a rapid surge in hormones that can make us very emotional and play havoc with our sleep, and are very aware of our developing sexuality and social relationships. No wonder that our teenage years can be such a difficult time to manage. Perhaps it would have been easier if we had evolved like butterflies, whose caterpillars disappear into a chrysalis to mature and emerge a couple of months later as fully grown adults! Sadly, this isn't the case – in fact, the transition is getting longer: in Western cultures at least, puberty is beginning at a younger age, but we don't grow into our final physical state of development for at least ten years from then. That is a pretty long time, and, given the various factors that can affect our eating, it is not surprising that many of us struggle with our relationship with eating during and after adolescence.

Understanding our emotions

All organisms have motivations to survive and reproduce. One way of thinking about emotions is that they are a way to give us signals that we are succeeding or failing in these basic tasks of life. They help us to attach meaning to events and relationships, and to recognise the things that we need. In his book *The Compassionate Mind*, Paul Gilbert outlines how we have evolved at least three types of emotional system. Each of these systems involves specific types of emotion, attention, thoughts and behaviour that can be very helpful in guiding us to meet the challenges of life:

- The first system is linked to detecting and dealing with threats, and so involves emotions like anger, anxiety and disgust.

- The second system is linked to detecting and responding to good things, such as food, friendships and sexual opportunities; it is linked to our drive to achieve and feelings of pleasure.

- The third system is associated with calm and contentment; it is linked with feelings of soothing, safety and peace, and also compassion and connection with others (affiliation).

These systems, and their key characteristics, are shown below.

Figure 3.1 Three emotional regulation systems

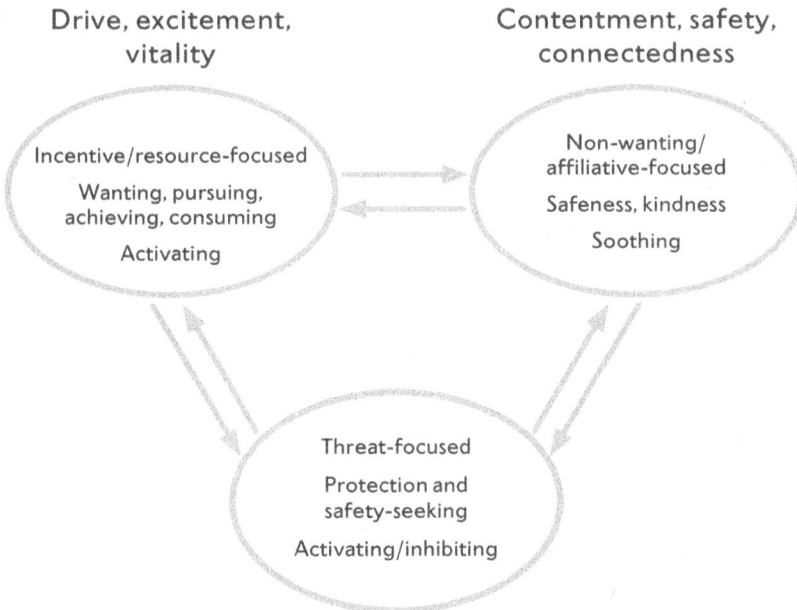

Drive, excitement, vitality

Contentment, safety, connectedness

Incentive/resource-focused

Wanting, pursuing, achieving, consuming

Activating

Non-wanting/ affiliative-focused

Safeness, kindness

Soothing

Threat-focused

Protection and safety-seeking

Activating/inhibiting

Source: Adapted, with permission, from Gilbert, P. (2009) *The Compassionate Mind*. London: Robinson.

The threat system: emotions of danger and protection

We are far better at detecting and responding to unpleasant emotions than pleasant ones. This makes a lot of sense because, during the time we were evolving, like all animals, we needed to detect threats from other animals (or humans) or from our environment (such as poisonous foods). The threat system is set up to work on the 'better safe than sorry' principle. Imagine an animal eating in a field that suddenly hears a noise behind it. The best thing to do would be to run away, to assume that the noise came from a predator. Nine times out of ten there will turn out not to have been a threat at all, but if this 'risk averse' strategy makes the animal run away the one time it needs to, it will save its life.

So, strange as it may seem, our brains are designed to make mistakes. They attach meaning to events rapidly and make us act quickly, a 'better safe than sorry' approach. This design also affects our memory and the things we brood on. Imagine you go shopping and nine shop assistants are very helpful, but one is rude. Which one would you brood on and talk to your friends or partner about? Most likely the rude one! And we will forget the 90 per cent we encountered who were actually kind to us.

Another difficulty with the threat system is that it is designed to overrule positive emotions. So, for example, imagine you're having a good time at a party when your mobile phone rings to say that your friend or child has had an accident. Or imagine that you're having a nice picnic on a sunny day in the park when you suddenly notice a swarm of bees approaching. In these situations, positive emotions are quickly turned off and you switch your attention to dealing with the threat. This is why sometimes when we are stressed it's difficult to engage positive feelings; as they can be suppressed. This doesn't always happen, of course, because some kinds of threats or risks are felt to be exciting – parachute jumping, for example – but the key thing here is that we feel in control of the risk or threat, so that we notice the 'drive' (excitement) emotions more than the 'threat' emotions.

What is very relevant to us here is that some people, when they are under stress, can actually try to turn off threat emotions by activating the drive system, or by using 'comfort eating', a regulator of the threat system! We will explore this in more detail in a moment. This threat detection and protection system is associated with rapidly activated emotions such as anxiety, anger and disgust, and defensive behaviour such as the 'fight or flight' response, avoidance and submissiveness. It is very easy to turn on, comes with powerful emotions that are difficult to ignore and can be hard to turn down – after all, we would not want a fire alarm that is hard to hear! It tends to grab our attention with both hands, and can be switched on by real events, memories and even our imagination. For example, I have a bit of a fear of heights. Even if I just close my eyes and imagine standing at the edge of a cliff and peering over, I will get feelings of vertigo and anxiety, and a strong desire to think about something else.

This threat system has evolved over millions of years and operates on many levels, some of which we may not even be aware of (such as looking around the room for spiders if we are afraid of them). It is strongly influenced by our experiences, as we learn what a threat is, and what is safe in the world. It is useful in helping us detect both physical and social dangers.

Although the threat system can give us a hard time, it is important always to keep in mind that it was designed as a protection system – it is not our enemy. Once we understand it and begin to work with feelings of anxiety, anger or aloneness (or whatever feelings the threat system is 'feeding' us), we can learn to respond in ways that have fewer unwanted side effects and that help us to manage life's challenges. Sadly, many of us learn quite early in life to be afraid of our threat system and the emotions it arouses – for example, to be afraid of being upset, anxious or angry. This often happens if these emotions have been responded to in a threatening way by others (for example, if we have been told off for crying or been hit when we were angry). Even worse, we learn to experience the bodily sensations that are activated when we feel threatened (the thumping heart, the sweaty palms) as a threat in themselves if we do not understand them. We can also learn to associate other sensations (for example, hunger), or even our own body, with the threat, particularly if we are worried about our eating or weight. So, as you can see, the threat system is a pretty tricky emotional system for us to manage.

The drive system: emotions of achievement and excitement

The second important emotional system concerns emotions that give us a sense of drive, vitality and achievement. This is associated with anticipated pleasure and excitement. It has evolved to motivate us to do things and to actively engage in the world. We get positive feelings for doing and achieving things, such as passing an exam, going on a date with a new person, going to a party or winning the lottery. When these things happen, we become emotionally and physically activated, and often we have a desire to celebrate. When this positive feeling is interrupted or taken away – for example, when we experience setbacks or failures – we can experience this as a threat, and this in turn can motivate us to try even harder.

Let's think how this might work if we're trying to lose weight. We can often be excited by new diets and feel a great sense of achievement, even pride, when we lose a few pounds. However, after several weeks most of us will break our diet or not lose as much weight as we did at first. This can lead to our feeling disappointed, even angry with ourselves. We can become afraid of failing, and this may make us try even harder to diet – or lead us to give up. That, as we saw with Aoife in Chapter 2, can have the unintended consequence of leaving us feeling anxious, angry or even disgusted with ourselves. Clearly, no one would want to feel this way, so our fear of losing this sense of achievement can be a great motivator. Indeed, many diet programmes rely on this system and use rituals such as group weigh-ins to mark individual success. Of course, they do not intend for those who do not lose weight to feel bad, but this tends to happen anyway! This is not to say that these groups are not helpful, but they may be helpful for different reasons – for example, because they offer affiliation with others, compassionate encouragement and support from a group. These are benefits that belong to a different emotional system, as we will now see.

The affiliative soothing system: emotions of connection, comfort and contentment

Our third emotional system is related to soothing and contentment through our connection to others (affiliation). It is linked with the experience of peaceful wellbeing and feeling safe. For example, imagine a parent who, seeing that their child is distressed, is loving and affectionate, and hugs the child until they calm down. This very common event is actually extremely important because it tells us that humans, like other animals, can regulate their threat system, and the feelings of distress and anxiety it generates, by experiencing kindness, affection and compassion from others (and from ourselves). We now know that affection and kindness actually affect how our brains develop. There are special areas of our brain and particular hormones that respond to the kindness of others, and to self-compassion and self-kindness, and this helps to defuse a sense of threat. Indeed, perhaps one of the greatest sources of contentment is being with people you feel loved by, and under no particular pressure to achieve anything.

This type of positive emotion is a very different one from that gained by achievement. It can help calm down our threat detection and protection emotions, and manage the unpleasant feelings we can experience if our feelings associated with achievement are interrupted. This system develops in childhood in response to being emotional and physically cared for, particularly when we are upset.

Soothing and food

As we have seen, food can be a way of giving us reward or excitement, and these positive feelings can temporarily make us feel better. We can also learn to use food to soothe ourselves. Indeed, the soothing system can become very easily associated with food, particularly sweet foods, and we can learn to turn this system on by eating. This isn't surprising, given that our earliest experiences of feeding are often associated with care and affection. You can probably imagine that one of the reasons why we soothe ourselves in this way is that we can find it difficult to reach out to others and deal with our emotions in an open way (perhaps because we're ashamed of or confused by them). We might even find that we're reaching for the food before we've even realised that there is emotional distress in us. Also, if we tend to be self-critical and find it hard to be compassionate towards ourselves, then one way to tone down these negative feelings is to turn to food.

How are food and emotions linked?

There are several other ways we can learn to associate food and eating with our emotions. Positive emotions can become linked via a learning process psychologists call 'conditioning', which connects one experience with another. We all have foods that we associate with positive memories. For me it is the smell of baking and the taste of uncooked cake mix direct from the bowl before it gets washed up – linked to memories of cooking with my mum and grandmother as a child. Even thinking about the smell and taste of these foods while I am writing brings back a feeling of warmth, happiness and comfort; I start to salivate and feel the urge to bake a cake!

We can also be taught by others that certain foods or tastes are associated with having a good time or even with a certain social standing (for example, caviar), while other foods (such as chocolate) may have a more direct impact on our mood by increasing the production of chemicals in our brain that stimulate positive feelings.

We do not even have to eat the food to experience its mood-enhancing effects; just imagining a nice meal, or even the smell of cooking, can lead us to feel full. We can learn to associate food as a treat, a comforter or even our friend. If it is taken away, or even if we feel we will not have it for a while, we can experience cravings.

Let's just imagine that I tell you that you must finish reading this chapter before you can go to the toilet. Many people tell me that just imagining this makes them want to go to, even if they had no inclination before. (Don't worry, you can pee now if you want to!) So, thinking or being told that we are 'not allowed' to do something can produce the urge in us to do it even if we weren't thinking about it before. My clients tell me that this happens to them all the time around food. When they tell themselves they are not going to have a cake, they find that the urge to eat one becomes overwhelming. Indeed, we can take a great deal of pleasure in the craving for and anticipation of eating our 'forbidden foods'.

If we are made to do without these – particularly if we use them to soothe ourselves – we can become angry, upset and even anxious, and end up feeling rebellious and resentful. I was watching a TV programme on healthy eating recently and heard that men of my age should eat a lot less sugar – and, yes, you've guessed it: now I really wanted some chocolate and to tell the well-intentioned presenter to get lost! If we set these rules ourselves, we can get into a real pickle, wanting to rebel, but also beating ourselves up for being so weak as to give in to our cravings – we can't really win sometimes, can we?

There is also a darker side to the emotional associations we can make with food. We can also learn to view certain foods as rewards that we have to earn, or even punishments that we have to endure (like eating our greens). We can also teach ourselves, or learn from others, that certain foods are bad for us, even disgusting, and become very fearful of eating them, particularly if we are told that they will make us fat, unhealthy or even just out of step with current fashions.

The emotions affected by dieting

Many people begin to diet just because they feel they've put on a bit of weight and want to lose it. But others begin to diet as a way of managing past or current experiences. These may include losses or major disappointments, bullying, rejection and difficult relationships, which in turn may fuel a desire to be more attractive, or anxiety about health. And, as we saw in Chapter 2, restricting our eating, or even planning to, can have a profound effect on our emotions.

In the early stages of our diet, we can experience a significant lift in mood and energy. This can help us feel better and more confident. Losing weight, or even just achieving the aim of limiting our eating, can also help give us the positive feelings associated with the drive system. Many people who diet are also concerned about the negative feelings they have about themselves because of their weight or shape, or are fearful of the judgements of others. Setting out to change our weight or shape, particularly if the way we diet is seen by other people, can help us to feel in control of these concerns; it can also help to show other people that we can manage our desire for food and our eating. Planning to eat less can have a positive effect on our mood, as we anticipate the benefits this will bring us. It can also help to block out more difficult worries or concerns, by giving us something else to focus on that is more in our control.

So, there are many reasons why dieting can make us feel good. However, as we also found in Chapter 2, dieting tends to fail after a period of time – in part because of our body's need to eat, but also because dieting tends to create problems of its own, not least of which is the distress caused by having to be constantly vigilant about what we eat. Of course, many people who overeat do not diet, but even thinking about restricting eating leads to these effects on our mood.

My personal reflections on the link between my three systems and eating

You may wish to a pause at this point to think about the role eating has played in deliberately or accidentally helping you to manage feelings. You can use these questions as a guide:

- Does eating or dieting link to your feelings? If so, which ones does it help with (e.g. providing comfort) or help to tone down/turn off (e.g. specific emotions like anxiety, disgust, sadness or combinations of different emotions)?

- What are your biggest worries about not using food to help with your emotions in the future?

- What would you need to work on to move away from using food to help manage your feelings?

The social and emotional influences on overeating

As we have seen, eating plays a big part in our social lives. Sometimes we will eat less in the company of others, but at other times more (especially if the occasion involves alcohol as well as food). So social pressure can go either way: to moderate our eating or encourage us to 'have another helping'. We can find it more difficult not to overeat when we are in bigger groups, particularly if we eat as a way of celebrating or belonging (note that excitement/drive system). Indeed, we can find ourselves eating more than we need to in order to go along with others and 'fit in'.

Many of us will know people who encourage us to overeat. They may do this for a range of reasons, including using food to show their love and affection, because they feel we are undernourished, or because they see making us eat as some sort of competition or battle, even as a way of keeping us dependent on them. Supermarkets and television advertising put a great deal of pressure on us to eat more. Many food manufacturers have increased their portion sizes over the years and increased the amount of sugar and fat in our foods, and 'two for one' and 'eat what you want' promotions are common. In fact, everywhere you look you can see encouragements to overeat.

People who overeat also tend to be less aware of the messages their bodies give them about when to eat and when to stop. Again, our changing social lives can make it even more difficult to notice these messages. Food tends to be eaten on the go or in front of the TV, and for many of us eating has become a mindless activity. Drinking alcohol while we eat can also distract us from the signals our body is trying to give us that we have eaten enough.

We have also become a less active society. Many of our jobs do not require much physical effort nowadays, but we are neither eating less, nor doing more activity in our leisure time, to take account of this. If anything, we tend to consume more calories as a society than we used to. We now live in a 'super-size' culture, less in touch with our body's signals and having been taught that we should want more than we actually need. All of these factors can play a role in patterns of overeating.

Attempts to 'solve' this problem have centred on the rise of the diet industry, coupled with the belief that being overweight is both a moral and a medical problem. People who are even a little overweight are often demonised. The weight fluctuations and dietary habits of celebrities can be a source of gossip and scorn. Jokes about people's weight are socially acceptable, as is the very real discrimination that overweight people can experience. It is not surprising that many of us will diet to lose weight, or just feel so bad about our bodies that we can't see the point in doing anything to improve our health or eating. Sometimes we can even overeat to punish ourselves for being in some way morally inadequate because we cannot meet society's expectations about what our bodies should look like. It is very sad that our children are not immune to these pressures. Their problems with eating can often begin very early in life. Children of eight, or even younger, can feel bad about their bodies and eating, even if they are perfectly healthy, at a normal weight and eat what they need.

Sometimes overeating can be a form of rebellion against these social pressures. We've already noted that many people diet as a way of managing difficult experiences; for a smaller number of people, overeating may be a way of trying to deal with painful events in their past, such as physical, sexual or emotional abuse, bullying or bereavement. A research study I was involved in suggested that at least half the people who come to NHS weight loss clinics are experiencing a degree of psychological distress that would warrant professional treatment. These problems included depression and anxiety but also worries about size and shape at levels similar to those found in clients with a diagnosis of an eating disorder.

Being distressed, for any reason, can make it more difficult for us to control our eating, even if we are not limiting our food intake. Overeating, or even anticipating overeating, can actually help us to cut off from some of our emotions, and may even give us a sense of pleasure that we may not be experiencing elsewhere in our lives.

Overeating, rules and self-criticism

Many people who overeat have a lot of personal rules about eating. These tend to develop over time and relate to their own personal histories and hopes and fears. Some are driven by fear that something bad will happen when they eat; others are based on the hope that eating will help them in some way. Other rules are learned directly from the messages with which the media bombard us every day.

These rules on their own are unlikely to motivate us to comply with them, so we tend to associate them with either a good or a bad outcome (such as 'If I overeat people will think I am greedy' or 'If eat less I will be healthier'), and with high levels of emotion (such as fear of failure or anticipated pleasure from achievement). Rules can also conflict with one another, leaving us very confused about how to behave!

Often, we are not aware of these rules until we break them. When this happens, we can be overwhelmed with a rush of emotion, often accompanied by anxiety-provoking thoughts, images or memories. Our rules tend to be plausible, even if we often exaggerate the consequences of breaking them. They will make sense for us, because they are based on our personal histories and hopes for the future, and it can be very hard for any of us to be rational about them when we are caught up in the strong feelings they are linked with. It takes a very brave person to ignore their rules to test whether their predictions of what will happen then really come true.

In Chapter 9 we will explore your own rules about eating and how you respond if you break one. For now, we will look at how these kinds of rules can affect various individuals' eating and emotions by looking at David, Jayden and Tomasz.

Eating rules in action

David is typical of many people caught up with rules about eating. He ate a reasonable diet and led a very active life, and his weight was stable. Then, sadly, he became quite ill. Over the course of the next year, he gradually put on 25 kg. He became very concerned about this and, as he recovered from his illness, decided that he was going to eat less. David set up many rules about eating, such as 'I must not overeat or I will get fat and have a heart attack or get cancer again.' His key message to himself was that if he did not keep to a very strict diet his illness would come back, he would never be able to work again and might even die. These thoughts were frightening enough to motivate David to limit his eating and he very rapidly lost weight. As time passed, though, he had strong urges to overeat and broke his diet. Full of self-recriminations, he forced himself back on to his diet until the same thing happened again. David followed this pattern of yo-yo dieting for the next ten years.

Sadly, Jayden had a difficult upbringing. They lost their father at an early age and did not find it easy to make friends. They found that eating could be a comfort and gradually came to believe that only food could make them feel better. Jayden had a lot of rules about when they should eat, such as 'I must eat when I want to or I will go crazy' and would often hoard food to make sure that they never ran out. They feared that if they could not eat when they were upset, their feelings would become overwhelming, and they would end up in a psychiatric hospital.

Tomasz told me that food was always used as a treat in his family. He was an only child and remembered with a great deal of affection how his parents and grandparents would always give in to his demands for sweets. There were very few boundaries, particularly around eating at mealtimes. He couldn't ever recall being told that he was not allowed to eat something the moment he wanted it. He had never learned to use his appetite to regulate his desire for food; instead, he believed that if he did not eat whenever he wanted to it meant he was being deprived or hurt in some way. Tomasz often got into a battle with himself when he tried not to overeat. He had two sets of rules: one was organised around the belief that he should limit his eating because of his health, the other around the belief that he should eat whatever and whenever he wanted, and if he couldn't do this it meant he wasn't caring for himself. The tension between these two sets of rules often led him to be very distressed when he ate anything, and he became critical of himself.

The idea of 'rules' sounds very formal, but all these rules are tied up with important emotions. For example, because Tomasz had never been limited in his eating, the emotions he associated with limiting his food were those of deprivation and a range of other painful feelings, including anger, frustration and helplessness, making it very difficult for him to see and experience taking control of his diet as being kind and helpful to himself.

It can be helpful to identify the rules that govern our eating, and to think about whether they are ones we want to continue to live by. It is important to remember that we are not always aware of the rules we follow in life unless we break them in some way. Some can be very helpful in keeping us safe and making life more predictable (e.g. driving on the correct side of the road for the country you are in), but this can become unhelpful or even dangerous if we follow them too inflexibly (e.g. driving on the left when the convention is to drive on the right). Even if we know we need to change our rules, we can often follow them by habit – which is why ferry terminals from Europe to the UK (where those driving rules differ), and the surrounding roads, have lots of signs about which side of the road to drive on! Even if we think it is helpful to change our rules about eating, this can take time and regular practice before a new habit forms.

My personal reflections on my rules about eating

Please write down any personal rules you have about eating.

- Where do these come from?

- Do they help you manage eating now?

- Does sticking to your rules come with any costs to you, or the people you care about?

- What (if anything) concerns you about breaking these rules?

What are shame and self-criticism?

The emotion of shame is a common risk factor for developing, and continuing to struggle with, eating difficulties. This can be what is known as internal shame (seeing ourselves as flawed, inadequate, inferior, powerless or personally unattractive) or external shame (believing that others see us as being flawed, inadequate, worthless or unattractive). Often these two versions roll together and are very painful. Humans will do almost anything to avoid them or turn them off. There are many routes into shame, including experiences of being excluded, bullied, humiliated, abused or not experiencing caring and validation. This is another powerful 'threat' emotion that our relationship with food and eating may help us with. It can lead to trying to lose weight, hiding behind a larger body than our natural set point or avoiding eating with others.

Shame and self-criticism often go hand in hand. People with eating difficulties tend to be highly self-critical and experience high levels of self-directed hostility. Like shame, there are many routes into self-criticism. One way to spot self-criticism is to note the way that we talk to ourselves, particularly when things are not going well. We can become angry, shouting and even swearing at ourselves.

We may learn to be self-critical because we are taught this by other people, or it may arise from frustration and anger at ourselves if we feel we are not living up to the standards that we (or other people) set for us. We may do this because we think it might motivate us to do better, or as a way of venting our frustration. Sometimes it can be a way of protecting ourselves – as we can think our own criticism will be less damaging and hurtful than criticism or disapproval from other people (by the way, we are usually wrong about this as our self-critic knows more ways to hurt us than anyone else!). Sadly, sometimes we can treat ourselves with feelings of disgust, hatred and anger, and may even use food to punish ourselves. Our self-critic can change over time, initially having the benign intention of trying to improve or help us but becoming increasingly hostile as we fail to meet its expectations.

Humans are not born with a self-critic or sense of shame – just the capacity to develop them. It takes the ability to think about our actions and our impact on the world around us before we develop this capacity (usually around the age of eighteen to twenty-four months). We tend to think that anything that goes wrong in the world (for example, our caregivers being upset) is our fault, because, if it is, we can do something to fix it. Self-criticism is absolutely not our fault, and we all do it, but it is something we all have to learn to understand and manage, as our tricky brains will do this to help us get a sense of control over things that feel out of control. One task of child-rearing is to help our children understand that they are not responsible for everything that goes wrong, and that there are things they can't fix (like me coming home grumpy after being stuck in traffic). Sadly, this tendency can be exploited by other people who would prefer us to take the blame, rather than admitting their own mistakes, or as a way of bullying or controlling us. This is a common pattern in many cultures, too, which tend to blame individuals or groups for social unfairness, discrimination, economic inequalities, or even the mental and physical health issues they can lead to. The compassionate mind approach was developed specifically to help us with shame and self-criticism.

Rules and self-criticism

You can see that David, Jayden and Tomasz didn't create the difficulties they experienced around eating; they arose as a consequence of their personal experiences and attempts to manage their lives in the best way they could and were certainly not their fault! Their stories show how our relationship with food can be affected by social and emotional factors, and how we can develop a lot of rules to help us manage.

Rules can be a helpful guide; indeed, without them, life would become very chaotic and unpredictable. The problem is that if they are too rigid, we are likely to break them. This can cause us a great deal of distress, as we can be very self-critical of our inability to keep to them. This is often because we are trying to encourage ourselves to do something that we believe will help us to feel better, so we see it as a sign that we are weak, bad or inadequate.

Marie was typical of many people who overeat. Although not actually dieting, she had two competing rules about eating. The first was that she should keep strict control over sweets or other 'junk' food or she would become fat and be bullied like her sister was. However, she also believed that chocolate helped her to feel better if she was upset. So, she spent her time oscillating between avoiding and craving sweet food. She allowed herself to eat it to fit in (for example, if someone brought a birthday cake in to work) or if she felt low, but her initial experience of pleasure through eating was rapidly washed out by the shame and guilt associated with breaking her rule. She tended to call herself names, and would feel disappointed, angry and even contemptuous of herself. She would then become self-critical and tell herself harshly to 'get back on the straight and narrow'. She often became angry with others for tempting her, and with herself for being so weak. Occasionally she would get sick of her rules and have a 'stuff it' day when she ate as much chocolate and as many sweets as she wanted, to help her deal with the misery of daily resisting temptation.

Marie was caught between two parts of herself: one that was condemning and critical, and one that was angry and rebellious.

These would battle it out – and neither of them was particularly helpful to Marie as a whole. Happily, she found a more helpful way of dealing with this conflict – by learning to pay attention to a third aspect of herself, which was compassionate, understanding and kind. In this way she could escape from the constant see-saw between being forced into change by self-criticism and self-dislike and being pushed into breaking out of her restrictions by feelings of anger and rebelliousness.

My personal reflections on Chapter 3

You might find it helpful to write down your key personal learning points from this chapter to help you find your own answer to what has influenced the way you eat now.

SUMMARY

As we have seen, the relationship between our emotions and food can be very complex. We can learn to experience positive emotions because of the foods we eat, or the associations we have with eating or not eating; and our culture and social environment can also prompt us into overeating. We can also learn to attack ourselves for the relationships we have developed with food, particularly for overeating, and this self-criticism can in turn make us overeat even more.

In the next chapter we will explore how compassion for these dilemmas, and for ourselves, can help us to develop a healthier and less distressing relationship with food and eating. We will look at how to manage feelings of distress, how to deal with our desires, and particularly how to manage the self-critical spirals that many people who overeat find themselves in. We will also see how compassion can help us learn to resist the social pressures we all experience that affect our eating and help us with the struggle with food that many of us face.

4 The compassionate mind

In the previous chapter, we explored how our relationship with food and eating can be very tricky to manage. In the following chapters, we will explore this in more depth and suggest practical ways to develop patterns that will help us to manage overeating. Now, at this point you may have the urge to skip straight to Chapter 14 in an understandable rush to 'do something'. However, please do bear with me for just a while longer. We have already seen that people who have any kind of difficulties with food and eating are often very critical of themselves, and that this can make the problems worse. What we are working towards is a compassionate mind approach, which helps us recognise our self-criticism and to disengage from it. When we can do this, we are on our way to taking long-term responsibility for our bodies, rather than just criticising ourselves into short term-compliance with yet another eating plan!

To do this, obviously, we need to be clear about what we mean by 'compassion' and the 'compassionate mind' approach. So, in this chapter we will explore the nature of compassion itself. The chapters that follow will guide you through some exercises to introduce you to the skills and practice of self-compassion, before we move on to considering how this compassionate approach can be applied to your relationship with food and, specifically, to overeating.

What is compassion, and why is it important?

Many spiritual traditions have suggested that compassion plays a key role in our ability to develop happy relationships with other people and happiness within ourselves. According to Buddhist beliefs, more than two and a half thousand years ago, in India, the Buddha came to realise that our minds are often chaotic, under the push and pull of various desires and wants, and that these are a source of deep unhappiness. This is because we can't always fulfil them, and, even if we can, it doesn't always lead to good outcomes. As we have already seen, simply eating anything we want when we want (as is now possible in our modern environment) is a recipe for problems.

The Buddha's solution to such difficulties of wanting, craving and attachment to things was the development of two key qualities of mind. The first is mindfulness – the development of a clearer, more observant awareness of how our minds work. This includes understanding how our minds create different thoughts, feelings, urges and desires within us. By learning to 'pay attention', in this moment and without judgement, to 'stand back' from and observe the changing climates of our minds (with the arising and passing of feelings and desires, fears and hopes), we can gradually learn to see these patterns of feelings and desires for what they are, and as a result learn to make better choices about what we do: which feelings we will act on and which we will not. There are now many books on mindfulness, and an increasing number of places where one can learn more about it and practise on retreats or under supervision. We will touch on the basics of mindfulness a little later.

The second key quality of mind identified by the Buddha, and the one that is central to our approach in this book, is compassion. Indeed, mindfulness is one way of developing compassion by helping us to recognise that some of our motives, intentions and feelings are not in the best interests of ourselves or others.

At its simplest, Buddhism defines compassion as openness to the suffering of ourselves and others, linked to a commitment and motivation to try to reduce and alleviate that suffering. In order to alleviate suffering, we need to understand its nature. The 'compassionate mind' approach taken in this book acknowledges a debt to Buddhist thinking and places these aspects centrally in its view of compassion. However, it also turns to new scientific thinking about our minds – how they work and are influenced by different processes that are linked to the way our brain has evolved.

The Buddha outlined a whole programme of living, which he called the 'Eightfold Path', geared to being compassion focused in the way we think, behave and act towards others. Now, the approach to compassion we're going to take here overlaps quite a lot with the Buddha's notion of the Eightfold Path, but with a very important additional aspect. This is rooted in the fact that we are all products of the flow of life on this planet. As such, we have evolved to need to be cared for from the day we are born to the day that we die. Feeling cared for by our parents, friends, lovers, partners and even our doctors, has a huge impact on how our brains, bodies and minds work. So does feeling cared for by ourselves – self-compassion. There is now very good research evidence showing that developing compassion for ourselves and for others is of great benefit to our mental performance, emotions, relationships, and our abilities to understand and cope with difficult feelings and desires.

Different states of mind

We've all had the experience of being in different states of mind – being angry or calm, excited or low. We can call an overall state of mind a 'mindset'. For example, we can be in a compassionate or a threatened mindset. The type we are in will affect a whole range of ways in which our minds work. It will direct our attention, focus how we think, urge us to behave in certain ways, texture the emotions that flash through us, influence what we're motivated to do and even affect the things we fantasise, dream or ruminate about. To show how this works, Figure 4.1 sets the threatened mind alongside the compassionate mind.

Figure 4.1 Two types of mind

Threatened mind   Compassionate mind

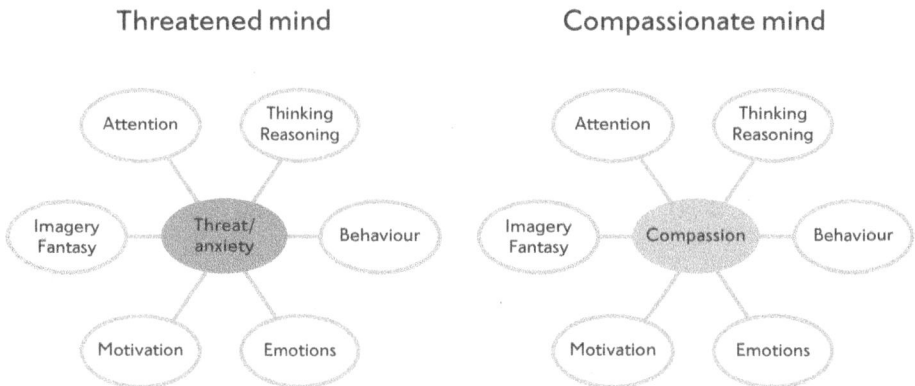

Source: Adapted, with permission, from Gilbert, P. (2009) *The Compassionate Mind*. London: Robinson.

As you can see, the six bubbles surrounding the central bubble are the same in both cases; only the core is different. So, for example, the threatened mind will generate one kind of emotion, while the compassionate mind will generate another.

Let's explore the concept of different types of mindset, because it is a key idea in terms of learning to develop a compassionate mind. Imagine that you are going for a job interview. This kind of event is naturally likely to get your threat system activated. Remember, this is easy to activate, as it's there to detect threats and help you respond quickly to them or avoid them. So even before the interview our threatened mind is working for us – and it may well start to switch on an anxious pattern. Let's look at this pattern by going around the circle on the left in Figure 4.1, starting at the top left-hand bubble (Attention).

In an anxious pattern, what are the things we attend to and focus on? We may well be focusing on what the other people will be like. How will the interviewers be with me – will they be friendly or challenging? We might have intrusive images or thoughts about previous occasions, perhaps when things have not gone too well.

How are we thinking and reasoning? Are we reminding ourselves that we've prepared a really good presentation and thinking how impressive it might be? If we're anxious, it is more likely that we are thinking we might not come over very well, reasoning that we might not present ourselves at our best and that the interviewers might take a rather dim view of us; or that someone else is bound to do better than us and get the job. So, our thinking and reasoning are focused on the possible threats in the situation.

What about what our body wants to do? How does it want us to behave? Now, you may want to go to that interview because you need the job, because it would be a step up, because it means a move to somewhere you want to go – any of the potential pay-offs. However, another part of you would rather not have to face it and wants to avoid going. Indeed, if you suffer from a lot of shyness and anxiety you might even have not applied in the first place! So, when our threatened mindset is running the show, it can fill us with strong urges to run away or avoid things.

The emotions of this mindset can be simple or complex. If it is only anxiety we feel, then that is reasonably straightforward, but sometimes it's mixed with wanting to engage with the thing that frightens us, so that our positive desires are pulling against the protective ones of avoidance. Indeed, the more we want something the more anxious we often are. Sometimes we can be angry with ourselves for getting anxious – for example, getting annoyed or disappointed for feeling shy in certain situations. We can become angry with our anxiety because we feel that it's holding us back, or that we are somehow different from other people. You can imagine that this gives an extra stimulus to our threat system. We now have two threat emotions to cope with: anxiety and (self-directed) anger – certainly not a soothing mixture!

The same potential for conflict applies to our motives – our basic desires, wants and wishes. There can be two types of motive: one relating to our immediate feelings and circumstances (wanting to get away from this threatening situation) and another relating to the longer term (wanting a better future). Our immediate motivation under the pressure of anxiety may be to run away or remove us from any possible threat as quickly as possible. It's simply the way our brains are built. Afterwards, we may well feel sad, because we've missed an opportunity – and that can, once again, lead us into self-recrimination and self-criticism.

Last but not least are the images, fantasies and daydreams we create in our minds. These complete the circle, for they are linked to attention. When we become anxious, we may have fleeting images of anxious memories or future possibilities. For example, we might create a picture in our minds of sitting on a chair in front of the interview panel looking a bit dumb-struck and awkward, while the interviewers look at us with stern faces.

So, our threatened/anxious mindset pulls on different aspects of our minds to create a pattern – and the different elements of this pattern feed each other. For example, the images that we create in our minds will affect our attention, thinking, feelings and how our bodies work. The way we think and reason about what is making us anxious will affect our attention, feelings, motivation and behaviour. This is why we can call the whole thing an 'anxious mindset', because it is about many aspects of the mind working together – with a common single focus on trying to deal with what we perceive to be a threat. The fact that these elements can feed off one another is important: your thinking can drive your anxiety feelings and they in turn drive more anxious thoughts, all of which pushes you along the road to more overall anxiety. And all of this happens, remember, because of the way our brains have evolved to live in conditions very different from those of the present. Thanks to evolution, we have brains that are very tricky to live with today.

Fortunately, there is an antidote to the anxious mindset that we can work on developing: the compassionate mind. This is based on understanding and caring and therefore will be more likely to activate the third of our emotional systems, the 'soothing' system, which, as we saw in the previous chapter, is a natural counter to the threat system. The kinder and more understanding we are, the easier it is to tone down the sense of threat that drives this spiral of increasing anxiety.

As well as the more general types of mindsets, such as the 'threatened mind' and the 'compassionate mind', we develop more particular types of mindset in response to particular types of problem. Let's take a look now at some of the most common mindsets that develop around food and eating.

Food and our states of mind

The dieting mindset

If you have struggled with your eating for a while, it is likely that you have tried to change your 'see-food-and-eat-it' mind into a dieting one. The dieting mind has two elements: it tends to see certain foods both as desired and as potential threats, and it also tends to focus on the achievements that dieting will bring us. Thus, it tends to activate both our threat and our achievement/drive systems.

Food as threat

For most people who diet, the threat will be one of weight gain. This means that food itself becomes a threat because overeating interferes with the real or imagined positive consequences of controlling their weight, and the mind organises itself in ways to help avoid the threat that eating poses.

In this mindset certain foods in particular tend to be seen as threatening, because they have become associated with weight gain or triggering overeating. The threat they pose may be related to their calorie content or to other nutritional qualities (such as carbohydrate, fat or sugar content). However, the allocation of 'threat' is not always a purely logical decision: sometimes it is because a food makes us feel full up or we enjoy its taste, and we associate these feelings with weight gain or the risk of overeating, even if it is less likely to lead to weight gain than other foods we have eaten that day.

If you are in this mindset, you will learn to pay attention to food in ways that people who don't diet are not really aware of. You may know the fat, calorie, carbohydrate, sugar or fibre content, or glycaemic index, of the foods you eat or drink. You may also be very aware of the calories you use when you are active or exercising. You are likely to spend lots of time thinking about eating, and to have many rules about what and when you can eat. You are also likely to invest a lot of time and energy in finding ways to avoid overeating. These may include planning and being on a diet, joining diet clubs or programmes, and deliberately not going out for meals with other people. You may become acutely aware of your feelings of hunger, but you are also more likely to be preoccupied with the smells, tastes and textures of food. You may even dream about eating!

Your 'dieting mind' will also make it easy to remember and think about the problems that overeating may cause you. For example, it may call up painful images of being bullied, or concerns about your health. You may think that other people will notice and disapprove of your eating and weight; you may imagine that they think you are greedy or out of control; you may even spend a lot of time comparing how and what you eat to what other people eat – or constantly compare your body size with others, or be particularly attentive to 'how people look' in real life or in magazines and the media.

Achievement through weight loss

Most people in the dieting mindset will also become very engaged with their drive and achievement system. As we saw in Chapter 2, this gives us good feelings when we pursue things we want or succeed in getting them. When you manage to keep to your diet you can get a buzz of pleasure – your biological responses to restricting your eating have actually evolved to give you this boost to help you deal with famine, particularly in the early weeks of eating less.

We may provide ourselves with many opportunities to check on and experience this success, such as frequently weighing ourselves, sharing our dieting success with others, planning for the good things that we imagine will happen when we lose weight – for example, buying new clothes – even comparing our own success with the failed diets of others.

Of course, it is understandable that you want these positive feelings, and for a while they can even calm down your 'threatened' dieting mind. However, if you start to struggle to keep to your diet, if you feel low for some reason and resort to comfort eating, if you start going out more often and having a good time and eating more – or if you just get fed up and decide to rebel, then these positive feelings can quickly dry up. When we have tried for something and then fail or suffer a setback, the baulked drive system can switch on the threat system and in come all those familiar sinking feelings – disappointment, frustration, even anxiety.

So, then you criticise yourself and try to force yourself back on to your diet. And, lo and behold, if you have a few successes you start to feel better again, get that initial buzz again, and the self-criticism and self-dislike die down. But of course, it probably won't be any easier to sustain this time around – so you will experience setbacks, the weight creeps on again, as does the disappointment and frustration – and you're back on the merry-go-round.

You can see how these two aspects of the dieting mindset can work together in Figure 4.2 overleaf. So, although feeling good about achievements can be helpful, on the other hand we need to be very careful about relying on it.

Figure 4.2 The dieting mindset

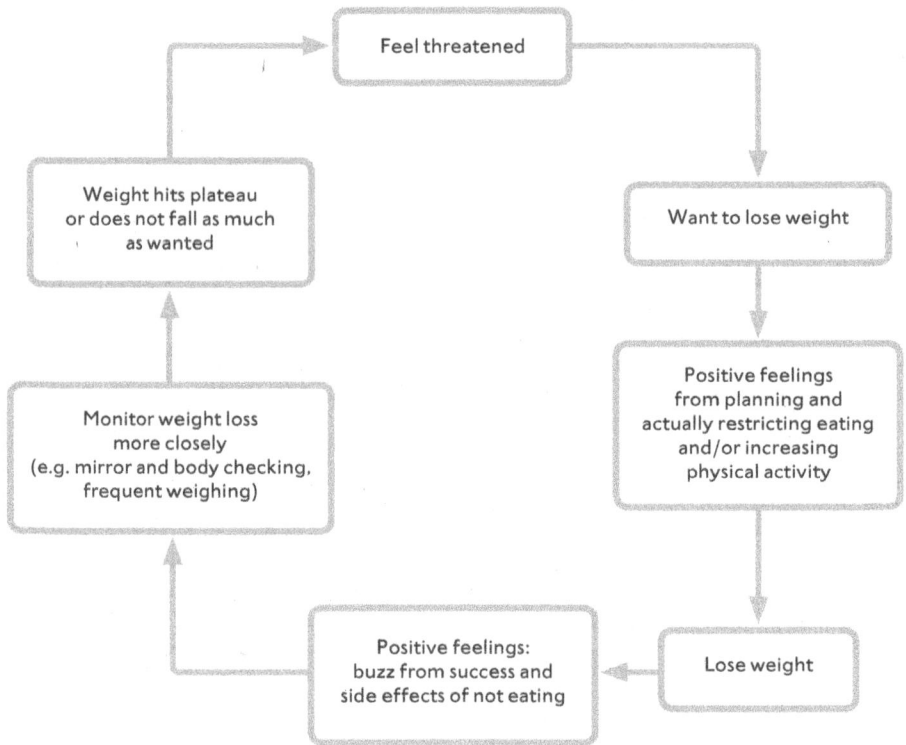

This can be one of the problems with slimming groups, which may overstimulate the drive system by being very positive about success and in so doing increase the chances of overeating or mood problems when people fail. It would be interesting to know, for example, how many people leave these potentially supportive groups because they feel ashamed that they can't maintain their weight loss targets.

The comfort food mindset

Another state of mind associated with overeating is what we can call the 'comfort food mindset'. This aims to help us with painful events, memories and feelings. You may remember that we learned that food is comforting from a very early age. The comfort food mindset also relies on the changes of mood, whether learned or innate, that we associate with certain foods. In trying to ease our distress, it draws us to the types of food and ways of eating that can either soothe present pain or block out memories of painful feelings. We can be preoccupied with eating as much as possible, over the shortest period of time, of the foods that will help manage our mood. This mindset can also involve a lot of planning, food shopping and arranging time and space (uninterrupted by others) for overeating. It will often remind us of our previous failed attempts to manage these problems without food. It will help you to override your sensory feelings of fullness and instead to focus on the emotional benefits of overeating.

As we saw in Chapter 3, our earliest experiences of eating (that is, suckling) are entwined and infused with feelings of emotional closeness, safety and comfort, as well as the physical alleviation of hunger. We can also draw comfort from what is called 'oral gratification' – the sheer taste and feel of those lovely foods in our mouth. What we want in this mindset is the comfort that comes from the process of eating itself, from the textures and tastes and the act of swallowing, rather than the feeling of fullness from having eaten enough. Comfort eating can help us to deal with a sense of threat, too, because if we're focusing entirely on the sensory experiences of eating, our minds are totally occupied and we can't focus on other feelings as well.

This kind of mindset is focused on the short-term alleviation of our pain and distress. Of course, in the long term it is likely to lead to a gain in weight and may not help us find other ways to manage the challenges we face in life. But when we are in pain, we tend to be less aware of these unintended consequences – or, if we are aware of them, we are so desperate to ease our distress that 'comfort eating' feels like our best option.

It is very common for this mindset to be linked to loneliness. When Carol began to monitor her eating behaviour, she noted that she tended to overeat in the evenings when her husband worked late and she was home alone watching the television. It took her a while to recognise that actually she was eating because she was lonely and trying to 'while away the time'. A deeper exploration revealed that, although she loved her husband, she felt somewhat dependent on him and had become rudderless in her own life, feeling that she was 'just drifting'. So, she decided that, rather than just focusing on her eating and waiting for her husband to come home, she would go and do some voluntary work on those evenings when he worked late. She found a group of people to join, which improved her social network and lessened her sense of isolation, giving her a purpose and raising her self-esteem. This is an example of where understanding what emotions are behind our 'comfort eating minds' can generate some very interesting solutions that actually have nothing to do with food. As we will see throughout this book, understanding our relationship with food often requires us to understand our relationships with ourselves and how the many facets of our lives interact.

For the moment, though, you can see that the 'dieting mindset' and the 'comfort food mindset' are both frameworks that our brains create to manage problems in our lives. It is really helpful to see that the way our brains do this – setting up patterns in response to challenges – is something they have evolved to do in order to help us survive and thrive. It's not your fault that sometimes, in the modern world, they actually make things more difficult for you. One of the problems in managing these types of mindsets is that they can exist in us at the same time. This can lead us into all sorts of tangles as we try to work out whether to diet or comfort eat, whether to diet to deal with the unintended weight gain that results from comfort eating, or whether to comfort eat to deal with the distress of failing in our diets!

The 'food as fun' mindset

Of course, we don't only see food as either threat or comfort. As we have seen, eating is often associated with sharing, closeness and having a good time. Being a good host often means providing food for people. There are countless books and television programmes dedicated to cooking and presenting aesthetically pleasing and delicious-tasting foods. There is no doubt that food can play an important role in a whole range of enjoyable social activities. So, we can get into problems with eating because we are just enjoying having a good time. We go to the restaurant intending not to have that apple pie after just having steak and chips – but everybody's enjoying themselves and we are one glass of wine the better, so what the hell!

We often feel our lives are so busy, hurried and stressful that we deserve a good time – we don't want constantly to be thinking about limiting ourselves or denying ourselves. We want to go with the flow and to hell with tomorrow. So, the 'food as fun' mindset is rather childlike, wanting to do as it pleases and have a good time.

This type of mindset is the one that starts looking forward to the weekend, to going out, to what you're going to eat and drink.

This is not about comfort eating; it is more about our drive/ excitement system taking over the show. You might also have noticed that this mindset can get quite irritable if it's told to fol- low limits and be quite resistant to any thought of constraint.

However, the *self-critical mind* (that is so strong a part of many of us who diet or overeat) can be especially down on the food as fun mindset the day after. We wake up feeling fat and bloated, maybe with a hangover to boot, and think to ourselves: 'Oh, why did I do that? Why don't I just have a little more control?' So, the self-criticism kicks in – until the next weekend, when maybe the rebellious childlike mindset says, 'To hell with it – let's have fun!' And so the cycle goes on.

The 'eat to fit in' or 'affiliative eating' mindset

This type of mindset centres on the positive feelings we get from our natural inclination to be part of a group. Sharing eating can help to bring our affiliative soothing system (which we explored in Chapter 3) into play. The combination of these feelings of belonging and safety with the physical pleasures of eating can be a really powerful factor in leading us into overeating.

This mindset can be associated with the 'food as fun' mindset, but this is not always the case. As we saw in Chapter 2, we can often eat to fit in with others. For instance, if people around us are eating a little less than we usually do, we will, unconsciously or deliberately, adapt our eating to fit in.

The reverse can also be true. In this mindset we want to fit in with others – so that we are seen as part of the social group, just to go along with the flow, or to make us appear desirable in some way. A good example of this in action is the business lunch or dinner. I have sometimes been out for a meal after a conference or meeting. Usually this is at the end of the day, when I have already eaten most of what my body needs. What I really want to do is have a light snack and go to bed. But out of my desire to be with people I like, or because I feel they will see me as impolite if I just slip away, I can all too easily end up eating a big meal that my body doesn't really want or need. And of course, if I have a drink or two as well, my resistance just drops like a stone.

Sometimes we eat like this to please the people we love – for example, if our partner has cooked a meal for us, even if we already feel full, we may eat it to make them feel appreciated. This desire to use food to cement social bonds goes back millions of years – but of course, our ancestors didn't find it so easy to feast as often as we do! This can lead to self-recrimination in the morning and activate the dieting mindset.

The 'food as punishment' mindset

This may be a little less common, but it will be familiar to some people. They know that the food or the way they are eating is not good for them but believe that they don't deserve to be treated any better; they may even use the food, or feelings of discomfort from overeating, to hurt themselves for some reason. Often people who struggle with this mindset have experienced traumatic or abusive histories and may need professional support to change this relationship with themselves.

An overview of our mindsets

We can see, then, that there are different mindsets – different parts of us, if you like: the 'dieting' part, the 'comfort-seeking' part, the 'let's have fun' part, the 'one of the gang' part – all of which (and you may well be able to think of others) have the potential to fuel problems with our relationship to food. Looking back to Figure 4.1, we can see how our different mindsets affect the way we attend to things, think about things, behave, feel, our motivations, and the kinds of images and fantasies we create. This is why we talk about these parts of us as 'mindsets', because they integrate different aspects of our minds. So, we also use the concept of a 'compassionate mindset' – or, for brevity, 'compassionate mind' – because it helps us to recognise that we're dealing with an integrated style of thoughts, feelings, how we pay attention to things, what we want to do and so on.

The other central point to remember is that these mindsets, which cause us difficulties with our eating behaviour, arise mostly because of the kinds of lives people lead in modern Westernised cultures – and I want to keep stressing this, for it is only in some parts of the world that it has become so easy to obtain foods that have been artificially enhanced in colour, taste and texture specifically to stimulate our appetites and to act as a source of comfort.

As we begin to understand in detail the key issues that lie behind our eating difficulties, we will come to see more and more clearly why we need to develop our compassionate mind so that, working with these other mindsets, we can take responsibility, with wisdom and understanding, for our own bodies – and learn to live contentedly and healthily with our 'see-food-and-eat-it' brain in our modern world.

Shifting towards a compassionate mind

It can be very helpful to become more aware of how our threatened mind works and, if we are overeating, to understand in particular our dieting and comfort food mindsets. As we become 'mindful' of these patterns and come to recognise how they are driven by the threat or achievement/excitement systems, we can also take steps to activate a different type of mind – one driven by the contentment/soothing system. This in turn can help us to learn to manage our 'see-food-and-eat-it brain' and to deal with the painful challenges of life and the pressure to 'just to enjoy ourselves regardless' or eat to fit in.

As we will see, the compassionate mind is never critical but always understanding of the difficulties of modern living and of the complexities and hardships we face. However, it is by no means passive. It is focused on and develops our inner wisdom. It is motivated to work in our best interests, to do things that are genuinely caring and to help us to develop a sense of wellbeing in the long term. Compassion takes the long view about our health and happiness, looking over and beyond just having a good time or eating to get rid of feelings on a particular day. It always seeks the 'middle way' and avoids rigidity and black-and-white decisions or behaviours – such as those inflexible dieting rules.

There is another reason why cultivating compassion is helpful and this is related to how our three emotional systems interact. Although, as we saw in Chapter 3, different types of feeling can sometimes coexist (we can be anxious and excited at the same time, or angry with people we love), harnessing one type of feeling tends to reduce feelings of other types – at least for a time. A group of psychotherapists called Behaviour Therapists (who focus on changing our behaviour) came to realise that we can learn to generate one emotion to dissipate another. They first focused on anxiety and suggested that the state of relaxation could not coexist with the state of high anxiety. This led to the development of relaxation training. So now many therapists teach anxious people ways to relax – and, indeed, help people to develop different feelings by creating certain states of mind

– through imagery, relaxation, body work or even dance. The point here is that learning to develop a compassionate mindset can reduce the power of our threatened, dieting and comfort food mindsets and help us to find other ways to deal with the challenges of life. Equipped with a compassionate mind, we are better able to take responsible and wise decisions that genuinely are in our best interests.

Our compassionate mind: an overview

Before you read this section, you might like to stop and look again at the outline of the compassionate mind in Figure 4.1 (see page 91). We are going to take a quick tour round that circle to see what each of the six 'skills of compassion' means in the context of the compassionate mind.

Compassionate attention will turn to helpful, supportive memories and a positive focus. Let's imagine that sometimes you overeat to comfort yourself for a lack of confidence; perhaps you feel uncertain about how other people see you or whether they like you. Your threatened mind will focus on the times when things didn't seem to go well (that's its job, of course, to bring the threat to your attention), further encouraging your 'comfort eating' mindset. Your compassionate mind, on the other hand, will direct attention to times when you have been successful, when you have got on well with other people, and will prompt you to remember when people have been kind.

Compassionate thinking and reasoning focus on understanding that overeating is a very common problem, and we all suffer from it to various degrees because evolution has given us tricky brains and bodies – not because of some moral failure on our part. It is also important to recognise how we can overeat either accidentally or deliberately, and how our biological impulses and responses around eating developed because they gave us an evolutionary advantage.

Compassionate behaviour is working out and taking actions that are in the best interests of ourselves and others. Sometimes this is fairly straightforward, but sometimes it may require us to develop courage and engage with things even when we are frightened of doing so or they are difficult. Compassionate behaviour might also involve learning more about our eating and practising different ways of coping with our feelings and nurturing ourselves. We can learn ways to manage our emotions and our 'see-food-and-eat-it' brain that will help us develop a healthier and happier relationship with food. It is very likely that we will need to develop compassionate behaviour 'one step at a time'. It is usually best to practise slowly and when it's easy to do so, to get skills in place before we need them. For example, if you're learning to swim, it's not helpful to learn in the open sea in a storm – far better to start off in the shallow end of a warm swimming pool! Sometimes it's hard to face up to things and so we don't practise and prepare ourselves. Compassionate behaviour is about kindly encouraging ourselves to do those things that are in our long-term best interests, even if it is uncomfortable in the short term.

Compassionate emotions are linked to feelings of warmth, support, kindness and belonging. If you try to give yourself encouraging thoughts, are you able to hear those in your mind with kindness and warmth? For example, if you're going to an interview and you think to yourself, *I have done this before, and if I don't get the job I'll be disappointed, but I can cope,* do you hear that in a genuinely kind and concerned tone, or in a kind of 'pull yourself together and stop being silly and getting into a state' tone? The emotions that we generate by talking to ourselves can affect how helpful our thoughts are. So, it is helpful to create compassionate tones and feelings in our minds when we are being supportive. The next chapter will introduce some exercises that, with the help of compassionate images, will enable you to practise this, and there are further exercises along these lines throughout the book.

Compassionate motives are at the core of our idea of compassion. These are the desire and intention to relieve suffering, and to behave in ways that genuinely enable you to flourish and support your own and others' wellbeing. Now, you might think that the best way to relieve suffering if you're anxious is simply to avoid the things that make you anxious. The problem is that this sets up another source of suffering, for if you have been anxious about going for something you wanted, then you have not been able to achieve your goal. Also, avoidance cuts down your options and increases the chances that you will feel anxious again. So, rather than learning how to deal with the anxiety, you get stuck with it. To make progress we have to be honest with ourselves: to really think about our values and the kind of person we want to be (or become), and how to bring that about, whether through tackling overeating itself or its consequences, such as weight gain.

Compassionate images are supportive, understanding, kind and encouraging. When we are anxious it is very easy to generate frightening or even self-critical images. But we can train ourselves to deliberately create different types of images in our minds and in this way stimulate different brain systems – especially the soothing/contentment system. Again, the exercises introduced in the next chapter will help you learn to create this supportive kind of image and to practise calling them up when you need them.

Our compassionate mind: the bigger picture

We are now ready to explore in a little more detail what we mean by a 'compassionate mind'. Why would we want to be compassionate, and where do our desires and abilities to be compassionate come from? The short answer is that they come from our motives and capacities to be caring. For example, as a species of mammal we give birth to live babies whom we look after and nurture. Evolution has given us protective and caring feelings towards our children. We enjoy seeing them grow and we become unhappy if they are distressed or hurt. Additionally, we have caring feelings for the other people around us such as siblings, parents, friends and colleagues. Their emotional states affect ours. We may even be affected by the distress or happiness of someone little known to us.

The reason why evolution gave us these motivations and feelings is complex, but basically it boils down to the fact that humans, and other animals that are motivated to help each other, survive and reproduce better than those who are not. This doesn't mean that at times we are not very selfish, critical and cruel – clearly, we have that in us too. It is our responsibility to understand these different potential states of feeling and thought and equip ourselves to choose which ones we want to activate.

Interestingly, it is usually when the threat system raises its head that we are likely to turn away from caring. We are less likely to have caring feelings for people we're frightened of, or who we feel are more powerful than us, or whom we don't like. Our attitudes towards these people are often wary and defensive, and that of course turns off our interest in compassionate caring. We fight our enemies rather than caring for them.

As we will see later, the same is true when it comes to relating to and thinking about ourselves. If we are angry with and critical of ourselves, that tends to turn off the caring and soothing systems that could help to combat the threat system.

As I have said, the reasons why these motives and feelings arose are complex; fortunately, we don't need to worry too much about their origins, apart from understanding that they evolved over many thousands of years. What we do need to do is understand them and then learn to harness them. So now I'm going to introduce you to the 'compassion circle' developed by Paul Gilbert (see Figure 4.3), who derived it from the research and ideas of many other people – including, of course, those from various spiritual traditions.

Figure 4.3 The compassion circle

Multi-modal compassionate training

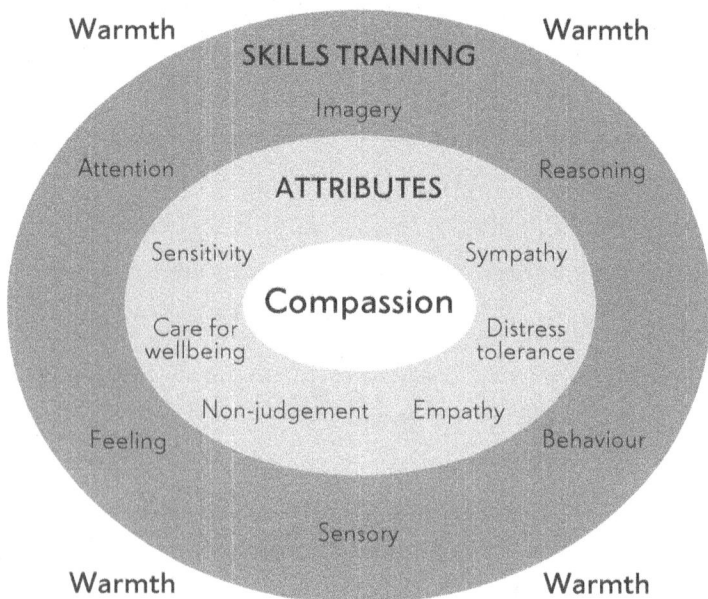

Source: Adapted, with permission, from Gilbert, P. (2009)
The Compassionate Mind. London: Robinson.

This model is based on the idea that compassion has two differ-ent components:

1. attributes that help us *engage with suffering*, in order to under-stand it, and this requires COURAGE

2. *wisdom* and *skills* to prevent or alleviate suffering, and these require COMMITMENT AND DEDICATION to learn and put into practice.

Compassion has four key qualities: wisdom, strength, warmth and responsibility.

Wisdom

This has two important aspects. The first is acknowledging that all of us simply find ourselves here, with a particular set of genes inherited from our ancestors and a very complicated brain that evolved over many millions of years – neither of which we designed or chose. The second is acknowledging that our sense of self and our memories come from our own experience of life, beginning with the relationships and situations into which we were born.

Our compassionate self understands this and acknowledges that while working with some of what goes on in our minds – powerful emotions, mood shifts, unwanted thoughts or images, and painful memories – can be difficult, there is no point in blam-ing ourselves for things over which we have had no control. We simply found ourselves here and have to deal with what we find as best we can.

Strength

This kind of strength is also called fortitude and is related to courage. It is not an aggressive power, but a source of inner confidence and authority that comes from wisdom. Strength helps to maintain our commitment and determination to face and heal suffering.

Warmth

The compassionate intention to relieve suffering is not cold or clinical but warm, friendly and gentle. This warmth is not (just) about being nice – it can be firm and persistent – but ensures that all its efforts are made out of a real desire to be helpful and not critical, soothing and not harsh, and are expressed in a gentle, friendly and open voice and manner. It is of course possible to act in compassionate ways without the feeling of warmth (for example, when we run into danger to help others, when we are feeling scared, or when we defend someone because we are angry); however, it can be a very helpful quality to address self-criticism or deal with setbacks.

Responsibility

Compassion is focused on facing rather than turning away from life's challenges. It involves recognising that even though we didn't cause many of the problems we face, we can still make a commitment to ourselves and others to do something about them, even if we work only in small steps. So, assuming responsibility is not about blaming or criticising but is about genuinely wanting to act in ways that are helpful and based on our wisdom, strength, warmth and desire to improve things for the future.

The full circle is given in Figure 4.3. OK, it may look a bit daunting, but in fact we've already gone through a lot of it. You see that the figure separates compassionate attributes (in the middle ellipse) from compassionate skills (in the outer ellipse). The attributes are the qualities that power compassion along, while the skills are the capacities that harness those attributes and through which they are translated into action. We will cover the skills in the rest of the book, so here we will focus on the attributes.

Compassionate attributes

Care for wellbeing

Let's begin on the left-hand side of the middle ellipse, where you can see 'Care for wellbeing'. This attribute captures the motivation to be caring; the decision and commitment that you wish to relieve suffering (in yourself and others). This might be a place to begin to look at the advantages and disadvantages of becoming compassionate: to think about what you have to lose in trying; to see if perhaps you feel you couldn't do it, so you've decided against it already – 'What's the point?' you say. Or maybe you feel that you have so many angry or other unpleasant thoughts and fantasies that you can't imagine being caring. Well, all humans have difficult feelings and fantasies, and this does not make you in any way less able to be caring, though it might mean you will need to focus on developing this attribute.

Sensitivity

Moving one place clockwise round the middle ellipse, we come to 'Sensitivity'. This means being open to what's going on in and around you; learning to pay attention and notice when you or others are in distress or are experiencing certain emotions. Sometimes when we feel distressed, we try not to notice it – because we 'don't want to go there'. Sometimes when we overeat, we don't want to think about the feelings that might be associated with what we're doing; or we might become angry with ourselves ('Oh gosh, here I go again! Why do I eat so much? What's the matter with me? Why can't I be like other people?!') rather than being sensitive, gentle and understanding. Many of us say unpleasant things to ourselves that we wouldn't dream of saying to another person who struggles with their eating. If we're honest, we lack sensitivity to our 'see-food-and-eat-it' brain.

Sympathy

Next around the circle is 'Sympathy'. Some people think this is a bad thing: it's like indulging, feeling sorry for or, even worse, 'pitying' yourself or others. That is a big misunderstanding. Sympathy is simply the ability to be emotionally moved by the pain of others or ourselves. Suppose you see a three-year-old child happily walking down the street. You may smile at their happiness – but then they trip over the kerb and bang their head heavily. Their laughter turns to tears as they experience real pain. You are likely to feel a flash of sadness and anxiety, and to want to rush out and make it better. Sympathy is that emotional connection to pain – it arises without thinking, moving us immediately. Developing sympathy for ourselves can sound more difficult, but it's the same principle. So, with wisdom, we can learn to be sensitive and open to our difficulties and also moved by them.

Distress tolerance

If we are aiming to cultivate sympathy and the ability to be moved by suffering, it may seem strange that we should 'tolerate' distress. In fact, this is a very important attribute. When the 'threat system' is in control, it pushes us into avoidance – away from unpleasant feelings. This is what it is designed to do; but if we always shy away from painful or frightening emotions, we never learn how to cope with them and the situations that provoke them. And the more we avoid them, the more we feel that we could never cope with them and so the more anxious we become. On the other hand, if we accept the difficult feelings – kindly, gently, uncritically – we learn that they are not unbearable and that there are ways to cope with them. So, learning how to tolerate our urges to overeat and our desires for food without acting them out (even postponing them for just a short time), and noticing how we can stay with our feelings, can be very important in helping us cope with them. Learning to be mindful and observant – having sensitivity – can help us with tolerating distress. Learning to be more empathic and less judgemental (the next two attributes) will also help us.

You can see how this works in practice if you think of a child who is anxious about going to a party with other children they don't know very well. Researchers have found that many anxious children have anxious parents who might let them stay at home, so they won't be anxious any more. Unintentionally they're teaching their child that painful emotions are not to be faced and dealt with but are best avoided. Because the child did not go to the party, they won't become familiar with the children they don't know, and so next time there's a party with those children, what are they likely to do? Yes – feel even more anxious and want to avoid it again. Sadly, while only wanting to protect their children, these parents are not helping them to understand how their minds work, or how to face up to and cope with difficult feelings and situations – which is a skill they will need in their future lives. It is tough to tolerate distress but, as you can see, compassion is not about avoidance – it's about doing those things that are genuinely helpful in the long term, and doing them kindly, gently and without harsh criticism.

Another reason distress tolerance is very important is because sometimes people think that compassion is about soothing painful feelings away – getting rid of them. Sometimes we can do this, but that's not always possible or even desirable. If we are very angry about something, we may need to learn how to deal with the anger: to be honest about our feelings and assertive. Compassion is not about avoiding addressing issues. Sometimes we have to learn how to tolerate powerful feelings and fantasies we don't like – even thoughts of hate. One of the biggest confusions and misunderstandings of compassion is the idea that it's simply about 'being nice' and hiding your feelings or suppressing them. That is not compassionate, and while brutal honesty all the time is not helpful, neither are suppression and avoidance. Of course, this is not an excuse to be rude or unpleasant, either. There are respectful ways to be assertive and powerful.

Empathy

Empathy is the human ability to think about and understand the nature of our minds and those of others. Unlike other animals, we recognise that people do things for reasons: because they are motivated, anxious or angry, because they want things and have desires, because they might not know the full picture – or because of impulses of which they're not even aware. We recognise that people can be mistaken in their views and have false beliefs. We can also reflect on how our own minds work. When we have empathy for our struggles with food and eating we're able to understand the nature of these problems, how they are rooted in the way our bodies and brains have evolved, how our own personal difficulties may have developed, what situations can make them worse, and the kinds of things we do when we feel the urge to overeat, eat unhealthy foods or restrict our eating too much. Empathy is a very important attribute in compassion because it is based on a deep understanding and acceptance of how our minds and bodies work.

Non-judgement

Last but not least is the attribute of non-judgement. This does not mean having no preferences or desires. Indeed, we know that some of our desires for food are inbuilt. Non-judgement really means non-condemnation; letting go of that angry desire to attack and be critical. The more we ease back from charging in and criticising, which can sometimes be our immediate reaction to a problem or perceived failing, the greater the chances we have for reflection and thinking about how best to deal with it.

How it all fits together

You can probably see from this brief tour of the compassionate attributes that they all build on and support one another. So, the more compassionate motivation you build up, the easier it may be to develop the other attributes. Equally, the more sensitive and the more empathic you become to your eating difficulties, whatever they may be, the more strongly motivated you will be to deal compassionately with them. In the chapters to come we will be working with this family of attributes to build up the overall compassionate mind approach.

We will also be working on the skills located in the outer ellipse of Figure 4.3. Like all skills, these are learned by practice: so, we can train ourselves in (for example) creating and building images that are helpful and compassionate, aimed at stimulating the soothing emotional system; we can train our reasoning and thinking to focus compassionately; we can train ourselves to behave in compassionate ways that are in our long-term interests. We can train our bodies to create compassionate sensations (for example, by using imagery), and we can use our images and other ideas to generate compassionate feelings. Last but not least, we can practise compassionate attention, looking for what is helpful and supportive in and around us, rather than letting the threat system always direct us towards the things we are frightened of or angry about.

My personal reflections on compassion

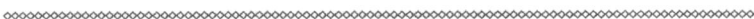

Sometimes when I introduce these concepts people tell me that they are not compassionate or 'can't do compassion'. I have never found this to be the case with the people I work with. However, they often struggle to recognise when they are being compassionate or believe it to be a superhuman feat in the face of extreme suffering. However, compassion is the everyday 'oil' for caring relationships and societies, and is something that can go by unnoticed and, often, unvalued in competitive cultures. In this book, my aim is to help you notice and use compassion in a mindful and deliberate way to make sense of your own suffering (including that which you may currently address using food), and learn to employ your wisdom, courage and skills to care for yourself and others.

Please think of a time when you noticed that someone was struggling with something they found a bit difficult or upsetting, and you offered your compassion, and they were able to accept this. Try to focus on something that has been resolved with a good outcome, and not a memory of something that is still currently difficult or very upsetting for you or them, as this may overstimulate your threat system. For example, it may be something as simple as someone not having the right change to get a supermarket trolley or someone needing directions. You might not have a recent example with a person in your life, so you could choose a scenario from a book or TV programme and imagine how you would be compassionate in that situation. When you have something that you feel is OK to work on, please try to recall which qualities of compassion you brought to the event (or that you imagine yourself bringing to the scenario):

* Which compassionate attributes helped you engage with and understand their suffering?

* What wisdom and skills did you use to help them address their suffering?

My personal reflections on Chapter 4

You might find it helpful to write down your key personal learning points from this chapter. This can help you to explore the key qualities and attributes of compassion that you may bring to help you address overeating, and the qualities and attributes you may wish to work on further using this book.

SUMMARY

By now you will have seen how our three inbuilt systems of emotions become involved with eating, and how complex these links and effects can be. Certain foods can be threats; losing weight can become an achievement that gives us good feelings when we feel in control – but then we can get into trouble if we 'lose control'. Eating can be a source of comfort or a way of rebelling against constraints and rules, a way of belonging to a group and even a way of punishing ourselves.

In the chapters ahead we will see how developing a compassionate mind approach can help us to deal with all these mindsets that can get us into problematic relationships with food. By way of preparing the ground, this chapter has provided an overview of how we see compassion within this compassion focused approach, and of the various elements that go to make up the compassionate mind. In the following chapters we shall be exploring all of these elements and how they can be applied to helping you to address overeating.

5 Preparing your mind for compassion

The previous chapter outlined the various aspects of the compassionate mind – a mind that is open to our suffering and the suffering of others and is committed to trying to reduce that suffering. A focus on compassion influences our attention, the way we think and reason, the way we behave, and our emotions and feelings. In the coming chapters we will explore compassionate ways of helping us change our relationship with food, eating and our body towards a healthier balance.

This chapter begins by helping you to prepare your mind and body for compassion by developing your ability to be more aware of how your mind is working and the capacity in your soothing system. These exercises are like physiotherapy for our brains, stimulating them in various ways. Just as our bodies respond to physical exercise by getting fitter and better toned, so research shows that developing our soothing system and our compassionate capacities can affect our brains, increasing our positive moods, and our ability to manage our emotions and impulses (for example, to eat). In later chapters, we work on developing our compassionate mind and use this to help us re-examine our relationship with food and eating.

As someone who has played a lot of sport and had a lot of injuries, I know that physiotherapy and exercises to get fit or develop sporting skills take time and practice to show their effects.

Progress is often best achieved by taking small steps rather than trying to do too much at once, and sometimes we need to strengthen certain parts of ourselves before we tackle anything more demanding. It's just the same with the exercises in this book: the more you practise, the more benefit you will get from them, but it's a good idea to take it slowly and not ask too much of yourself all at once.

As with any new skill, we don't want to practise under pressure. Ideally, try to practise when you are feeling relatively OK – or at least, not when you are really cross, miserable or frustrated with your eating habits. As you get better at using each skill you will gradually be able to incorporate them as alternative ways of managing discomfort or distress, instead of using food or being self-critical.

A 14-day soothing challenge

One way that you can use this chapter is to set yourself a 14-day soothing challenge to develop your mindfulness skills and soothing system. I would suggest giving yourself thirty minutes per day to do this. Once you have learned a skill, it may be easier to practise 'little and often' and to build it into your daily routine – for example, doing a couple of minutes of breathing exercises in the morning, or while walking or waiting for the bus. Imagery exercises require more time and a quiet place to do them, and of course you can do the more practical approaches to soothing for as long as you want. You can use the 14-day soothing challenge worksheet (pages 150–1) to set your daily goals, reflect on the exercises and choose which ones work best for you.

Choosing what we pay attention to

You may have already noticed that our minds can be quite unruly things. I am doing my best to concentrate on writing the next sections of this book, but I have at least three other things buzzing around in my head, including planning for the weekend, wondering what to cook for dinner, and the bill I need to pay by tonight! The good news is that this is perfectly normal; our brains have the ability to multitask. However, we can find it especially difficult to concentrate on one thing if our threat system is very active. In evolutionary terms this makes sense, as we need to pay attention to any threats in order to keep us safe, so the threat system has evolved to be very good at distracting us from anything else. These days, though, our feelings of threat are quite likely to relate to things that are not an immediate danger to our survival, and we need to learn alternative ways to manage them – including being able to focus our attention where we want it. This can be especially useful in dealing with impulses to diet, overeat for comfort or criticise ourselves for how we are eating.

We are now going to explore two ways of working with your attention. The first is to develop your capacity to be mindful of the thoughts and feelings that you experience. The second is to develop your ability to deliberately refocus your attention.

Mindful attention

There is a very long tradition in Eastern religions, particularly Buddhism, of training attention. The practice of doing this is known as 'mindfulness'. In recent years, therapists have discovered that learning to be mindful is extremely beneficial for a range of psychological difficulties and in dealing with the everyday stresses that all of us face. Mindfulness is a way of paying attention to the things going on around us and in our own minds. The aim is to be fully in the present in each moment, rather than constantly being pulled away with worries, plans and ruminations. Learning to recognise when we are shifting away from the present moment and then returning the attention to our desired focus is the key. Mindfulness is not 'making' your mind pay attention or emptying your mind of thoughts – it is noticing the shifting of your mind and then returning it to its focus. As we will see later, this can be very helpful when doing compassion exercises.

A second aspect of mindfulness is noticing how our thoughts and emotions emerge – for example, learning to pay attention to the bodily experiences of wanting to eat and to label them. So, we might say to ourselves: 'I'm having the feeling in my body of wanting to eat; I am having fantasies of biscuits and chocolate cakes; I'm feeling the urge to put those in my mouth.' In this way, the feelings are no longer just semi-conscious impulses guiding your behaviour. By bringing them into the forefront of your consciousness and paying them attention, you learn to observe them and really know what they feel like. Learning to 'speak the feelings out' like this – putting words to our thoughts, feelings and fantasies – helps us to slow down and to become more aware of things emerging in our minds and bodies rather than just following our impulses.

You might also become aware that when you try to resist the urge to eat, another set of feelings, urges and thoughts will appear in your mind, which try to nudge you towards overriding that resistance. These would include the 'stuff it' thoughts, such as 'Oh, stuff it, I want to eat and I'm going to!' or 'Stuff it, I don't want to think about this and I'm just going to eat!' You might then follow that thought curiously and wonder where it's come from, what it's about and what happens if you challenge it. Or, if you have feelings of anxiety about eating, when you become mindful you will pay attention to the anxiety as an observer and again be curious about the thoughts that pop into your mind as a result.

So, to be mindful is to become more observant of the ever-changing flow of emotions and thoughts that ripple through our bodies and pop in and out of our minds. Once we have learned to observe these, we can begin to make choices about whether to act on them or not. So, the key to mindfulness is this slowing down, paying more attention to the present moment and becoming more observant of the contents of our mind and the feelings in our body. We will explore this approach in Exercise 5.1, but first we'll take a brief look at another way of training our attention.

Refocusing our attention

This is somewhat different from mindfulness. It involves learning to use imagery or physical activity deliberately to shift our attention away from the present to a mindset we would prefer to be in. Like summoning up fleeting images, this is something that we do naturally and voluntarily – for example, all of us have probably chosen to daydream about our holidays to take our mind off some rather humdrum or unpleasant task, or to do something that we know will distract us from thinking about something difficult. Later in this chapter we will look at how you can learn to refocus attention to get yourself into a specific mindset, when we explore the idea of a 'soothing place', and we will also use this skill in the next chapter to develop compassionate imagery.

Exercise 5.1: Mindful attention

Please sit quietly for a moment and focus on your breathing. Allow the breath to come right down into your lungs slowly and evenly, and then leave your body slowly and evenly. If you find this difficult, you may simply want to try to focus on the sensation of your breath coming in and leaving through your nose. Try spending two minutes simply holding your attention on the experience. If you don't like focusing on your breathing, you could focus your attention on looking at and feeling a pebble or a shell.

You may notice that within just a few moments your mind will have wandered off on to something else. This happens to all of us: we all have things in our minds, and our attention easily gets pulled towards them and away from the present moment. It happens whether they are things that are worrying us (an interview coming up), that we are looking forward to (like a party), or that we need to do (pay a bill or remember to call a friend) – our attention will skip from one to another. This is absolutely typical of how our minds work; indeed, recent research evidence suggests a 'wandering mind' is our natural state.

One aspect of practising mindfulness is just learning to notice when your mind wanders, and bringing your attention gently and warmly back to what you want to focus on – that is, not beating yourself up for having a wandering mind but kindly and uncritically pointing your attention back to the moment. Telling ourselves off for not being able to pay attention is not being mindful! Indeed, this self-criticism is counterproductive, as it can actually be very useful to notice where your mind wanders off to, as this will often help you to identify issues that are bothering you and prompt you to do the work needed to resolve them. The very fact that you find this difficult is itself evidence that you are engaging in mindful practice.

You might try to practise this 'mindful attention' exercise for a couple of minutes, three times a day. In the early stages you may only be able to focus your attention for 10–20 seconds at a time. That's fine. Remember, the key is to notice where your mind wanders to and gently bring it back to the present moment, focusing on your breathing, or your shell or pebble.

Developing our mindful attention skills can provide us with a useful way to slow down the rush to follow our impulses to eat and help us to notice what drives them. However, it can be helpful to have a structure for eating in place before applying mindfulness to the experience of eating, and so we will postpone exploration of eating mindfully until Chapter 15.

What is soothing?

Soothing is the pleasurable experience of feeling peaceful contentment with a calmness of the body and mind. It is also linked to a reduction in physiological arousal, such as a slowing in our heart rate, breathing and stress hormones. It is associated with physical and mental wellbeing. Soothing can occur if we are in caring relationships (with humans or animals) but we can also learn to stimulate it on our own. It can help us feel more connected to others and is often used in therapy as a bridge to our compassion system. Soothing is different from distraction, which temporarily takes our mind away from threat, as we are actively trying to change our physical and mental state. Developing this system will change our brain to improve our 'window of tolerance' for threat, in other words how quickly and intensely our threat system is turned on and how quickly we are able to calm down after it is triggered.

Many people I have worked with find it difficult to turn this system on or can only do so by using food. In the rest of this chapter, we will explore different ways for you to do this as part of your 14-day soothing challenge, including practising ways to develop your soothing system, changing breathing patterns, imagery and spending more time being connected to people or animals.

Key to your challenge is to become aware of when you are in your soothing system, understanding what already helps you turn it on and experimenting with new ways to switch it on when your threat system is relatively small. Then you can deliberately use your soothing system to help you when your threat system is larger, to manage your urges to overeat.

Soothing and compassion

This book does not aim to 'soothe away' life's problems, difficult memories or emotions. To address these we need the wisdom, courage and skills of our compassionate mind (and sometimes the compassionate mind of others). We will use soothing to help you develop your 'window of tolerance' (your ability to tolerate distress and how quickly you can calm your body and mind), to help you change emotional 'gears'. We know that if we try to go straight from first gear to reverse in a car when we are still moving forward, we will end up with a loud screeching noise and a lot of our gearbox in the road! Our mind and body are no different. It is very difficult for them to move into a wise compassionate state when we are in a high state of threat. They need to calm a little so we can bring our compassionate capacities to bear on what is triggering or maintaining our threat system. Our compassionate mind can often change gears more quickly if we are caring for someone else, as this is what it evolved to do. However, this can be more difficult to do for ourselves, hence the need for our soothing system to help us. First responders know this and will often spend a moment regulating their breathing after a blue-light drive to an emergency. I also use soothing to prepare my mind for compassion when working with clients, particularly if I am going from managing a difficult email into therapy.

How does my soothing system work now?

The first step to developing your soothing system is to notice what you already do, and ideally to do more of it!

Please spend some time trying to recall when you have been in your soothing system in the last week that was not only related to the tastes, textures and quantity of food you have eaten. It is fine if this was around mealtimes, if you were doing something else or were with people or animals that helped you feel soothed. Write down anything that helped you feel soothed, even if this was only for a very short period. You might also find that some of the things we will explore as distractions in Chapter 8 also have the effect of soothing you; but please remember, soothing is not just the absence of threat – it is a clear change in your mind and body.

If you can think of anything that you already find soothing, plan to do this more often over the next week when you are not in a high threat state and make a note of how this goes so you can learn what works best for you.

Using our senses to activate our soothing system

Learning to use our senses, and mindfully focusing on our sensory experiences, can help us to activate our soothing system. Indeed, some therapy programmes use the experience of nature walks specifically to do this. Here we are trying to immerse ourselves in a sensory experience that helps us be calm and contented in a way that feels safe for us. It is likely that you will find that some sensory experiences do this better for you than others. Sometimes the experiences we focus on in our soothing place can give us clues to what works best for us. Play with all of your senses to find which ones soothe you. You may well find that different sensory experiences affect you more strongly at different times; this is perfectly normal.

In the exercises that follow we will explore how to use our senses of sight, hearing, touch and smell to activate our soothing system. Taste can also be a powerful way to bring our soothing system into play; however, as we are trying to break the association between eating and feeling soothed, it is more helpful to avoid this sense as a way to soothe yourself, at least until you are sure that it won't lead to overeating.

Whatever exercise you do, it is likely that your mind will wander. Just notice where it wanders to and gently return to the experience that you find soothing. If your mind returned to your threat system, this is perfectly normal – you might want to make a quick note of the themes your mind wanders to so you can work on these using your compassionate mind, when you are ready. There is often wisdom in our threat system that needs to be understood and addressed, rather than ignored or eaten away.

Soothing by sight

The things we see can be very powerful in triggering our soothing system. As with all the senses, to find out whether this works for you, try to immerse yourself in the experience and pay mindful attention to the things you can see.

In choosing what you find soothing to look at, take care to avoid anything that is associated with unpleasant memories or events. People I have worked with have found it soothing to look at a beautiful flower, a lit candle or a burning fire, an intricate shell or a smooth pebble. Alternatively, you may find it more soothing to look at a wider range of things, in which case you may want to visit a museum or gallery, sit in the lobby of a beautiful hotel, take a walk and look at nature around you, or go out in the middle of the night and watch the stars. Some people prefer to make their own scrapbook, or even to make one space in a room visually appealing so they can control the range of things they want to look at.

Soothing by hearing

We know that humans can be very sensitive to sound. Babies in the womb can be calmed by certain types of music or startled by loud noises. Again, the key is to discover the sounds that you find soothing and to be a little careful in what music you choose. Musicians throughout the ages have used music to create certain moods in us; so, to call up a feeling of being soothed, it's probably best to avoid loud, invigorating or sad music! Some people find the sounds of nature (waves, birds, rainfall or leaves rustling, for example) to be soothing. I personally find some voices comforting; you may find that a particular actor's voice does this for you, or the voice of someone you know personally. Some people I know use audio books to help soothe them; some even request my voice to talk them through the exercises we use in this book, while others prefer to have a friend they know and trust make a recording of the exercises for them to use. Other people prefer to record their own voice (particularly when they find a compassionate voice tone – we will explore this in the next chapter).

Soothing by smell

The fastest way to a person's heart – actually, their brain – is not through their stomach, as the popular saying has it; it is through their nose! Our sense of smell is our fastest-acting sensory system – which makes sense in evolutionary terms, as we can often smell danger long before we can see it or hear it, let alone touch it. You could use your favourite perfume or lotions, or you might find that natural smells are more soothing: you can experiment with the smells of different flowers, fruits or other natural products (like pine or cut grass). Many of these can now be found bottled online.

Soothing by touch

Touch can be a powerful source of soothing. Studies of infant monkeys found that if they were fed without comforting touching, they suffered serious difficulties in their development and grew up to be fearful. There is now a lot of evidence that affectionate touch has many positive effects on us. When we're anxious, being touched by another person who we feel cares for us can reduce our anxiety more quickly than even the most powerful anti-anxiety drugs. This is probably not news to you; it comes to us automatically to reach out and hold our children, friends or partners if they are in distress. The key here is to allow ourselves the opportunity to experience touch in a way that feels safe for us. This can include planning more hugs into your day or having a massage. Even if other people are not around, we can massage ourselves or even imagine being held.

Human touch is not the only tactile experience that can soothe us. Pets can have a similar effect; indeed, some hospital wards even have a 'therapy pet' system because stroking a pet can help soothe clients and even speed up the healing process. Even something that simulates the feel of a pet (for example, a fur-covered hot-water bottle) can be soothing for some of us.

Other tactile experiences that we may find soothing include smoothing a creamy lotion on our hands or body; placing a cold compress on our forehead; or even brushing our hair for a long time. Physical warmth can also be soothing – for example, having a warm bath, cuddling a hot-water bottle or sunbathing (don't overdo this, though, and make sure to put on some sun cream!). For other people, the experience of slipping into fresh, clean sheets or silky clothes, or sitting back into a comfortable chair, can be very soothing.

Please chose at least one sense per day and experiment with the things that may help you feel soothed by looking at, listening to, smelling or touching something, or having something or someone touch you. Make a note of how this feels in your body and mind. Once you have found what works for you, spend a few minutes several times per day repeating this experience when you do not feel too stressed. When you know this can reliably bring your soothing system online, you can experiment with which activity can help you when your threat system is online. You can of course spend longer in sensory soothing (for example, if you find a bath soothing you don't have to jump out after two minutes!). Remember that your wandering mind may pull you away from any of these experiences, and that you may need to gently refocus on the experience of being soothed.

Multiple sensory soothing

You may find that you prefer to be soothed by just one of your senses, or by a combination – for example, listening to soothing sounds while holding something warm and furry. The key is to be mindful of the experience and to allow yourself to take joy and pleasure from the experience. There is no 'best way' to do sensory soothing, just what is best for you on a given day. I would suggest keeping the things that you find helpful with you in some way. For example, I get quite stressed at airports so I make sure I have pictures of my family and pet to look at while listening to soothing music.

Some people prefer to take a more active approach to being physically soothed – for example, taking part in formal relaxation training, yoga or meditation classes. This is absolutely fine, as long as you find it activates your soothing system.

Part of your 14-day challenge is to practise your physical self-soothing skills every day. You may wish to draw up a list of the types of things you can try, and to practise each one for several days before moving on to try another. Over time, you will find your own menu of things you find physically soothing. Sometimes you can get the best of both worlds by using them while doing other soothing exercises, like soothing rhythm breathing.

Soothing rhythm breathing (SRB)

In the previous exercises you may have noticed that your breathing naturally changes when you are in your soothing system. In this section we will explore how deliberately changing the way you breathe can help bring your soothing system online.

Soothing rhythm breathing (SRB) is designed to help you find your own rhythm for breathing, rather than following a specific rate or pace, such as those suggested in some relaxation training or breathing apps. The main reasons for this are that we all have different lung capacities, and slightly different patterns in pace, depth and smoothness of breathing that we find soothing. This can also change over time, as we get more practised at feeling soothed. The key is to find a rhythm that you find soothing each time you do the exercise. If you find an app/recording that helps you keep to a rhythm that works for you, that is fine too.

Finding your SRB

Begin by finding a quiet place where you know that you will not be disturbed for at least ten minutes. Sit in a chair with an upright posture, don't let your head rock forward, and place both feet on the floor about shoulder width apart. Rest your hands on your legs. The key is to feel stable in your seat, your feet feeling grounded with the floor, with your head upright so that your breathing is not impeded by your torso being scrunched up. Please keep in mind that you are not aiming to 'achieve' any specific emotional or physical state in this exercise. It is designed to help you explore how your breath links into your soothing system and to see what happens. Training your soothing system to this posture can also be very helpful, because when you sit like this your body will remind itself to move into your soothing system, sometimes even without you deliberately changing your breathing.

When you feel ready, begin by gently focusing on your breathing. Initially just notice the breath going in and out though your nose. Notice the air coming down into your diaphragm (that's just at the bottom of your ribcage in the upside-down 'V') and how the diaphragm moves. Simply notice your breathing and then you can experiment with your breathing rate.

Now try to breathe a little faster than you normally would for 10–20 seconds. If you do not find this soothing, just stop and return to your normal rate for a moment. Then try to breathe a little more slowly for 10–20 seconds. Again, go back you to your normal rate if you do not find this soothing. Spend several minutes experimenting with these rates until you settle on one that works for you.

You can now try breathing more from the top of your chest for 10–20 seconds. Please stop if you don't find it soothing and return to how you normally breathe for a moment. You can then try breathing more from your abdomen for 10–20 seconds. Spend several minutes experimenting with the depth of your breathing until you settle on one that works for you.

The final experiment is to find out if irregular and ragged breath is more or less soothing than regular or smooth breath. Imagine you are a bit unfit and have run for a bus, then try to breathe like you would when you get on board! Try this for 10–20 seconds and notice how this feels in your mind and body. You can stop at any time if you don't find this soothing. Then try to breathe more regularly and smoothly for 10–20 seconds to see if you find this more soothing.

Even in the 10–20 seconds you were doing these exercises, you may have noticed that your wandering mind crept in with other thoughts, or that you became distracted by other noises in the room. When that happens, just notice that the mind has wandered and gently and kindly bring it back to its focus. At all times remember that you're not trying to force yourself to do anything, to clear your mind of thoughts or make yourself concentrate. You are simply noticing and gently refocusing, noticing and then refocusing. When you first do this, it can be quite surprising just how much your mind does shift from one thing to another. This is all very normal, natural and to be expected. You might notice, for example, that you feel your body becoming heavier in the chair. You are not trying to force your mind to clear itself of thoughts. If you have one hundred thoughts, or even a thousand, that doesn't matter at all. All that matters is that you notice, and then, to the best of your ability, gently and kindly bring your attention back to the breathing. If you use the motto 'attention and return' gently and kindly to guide you, you may find that your mind will bounce around less. It may become easier, but some days it will be easier than others. If you have thoughts that you are not doing it right or that it cannot work for you then note these as typical intrusions. Remember, the wandering mind can provide us with very useful information to work on later. So don't get angry with it, or become self-critical, just kindly bring it back to the focus of your breathing. It is the act of noticing how our minds wander that is the beginning of mindfulness.

SRB – anytime, anywhere

Generally, SRB involves breathing slightly slower, slightly deeper, in a more regular pattern and with a smoother flow of air in and out of your body than you would normally do (particularly if you are in your threat system). However, your SRB may change on different days. Over time, you will learn your 'range' and the SRB you need to turn on your soothing system.

You can try engaging in soothing breathing at any time and in any place, such as sitting on a bus. It just involves allowing yourself a moment where you focus on your breathing and for your mind to come back to that single focus.

Once you have found an SRB that works when you are seated, you can then try to do this standing up. Keep your feet hip width apart. This helps us to feel stable and grounded. You can imagine that someone is giving you a slight push from the side, then let your legs find a comfortable position to help you stay upright. Again, explore your breath to find what helps you to feel soothed; this may be different when you are standing up.

The final variation is to find your SRB then set off on a short walk while trying to keep this rhythm. This does not mean taking one step for every breath! Just see how it feels trying to walk and feel soothed at the same time. I sometimes use this approach to help me prepare my mind for compassion after a stressful commute. Many people who have tried this report that it helps them notice things around them, which can lead to further soothing using their senses. The key thing is our mindful attention to the process rather than the result. This is a bit like sleeping, where we try to create the conditions that will help us sleep, but if we focus too much on whether we are 'asleep or going to sleep' this makes it more difficult.

During the book we will use soothing to help you prepare your mind for compassion. However, you can use the exercise to relax and rest your mind or even help you sleep. Indeed, it is not unusual for people to feel very sleepy when they do SRB – it is our body's way of telling us we need to take time to rest and restore ourselves!

Working with imagery

Images can be very powerful and rapidly activate various systems in our brain. Certain images can stimulate the parts that help us to feel soothed and safe, and at the same time tone down other emotional systems (especially the threat system) that may be associated with eating difficulties. In this way they can help us to break the association between food and emotional comfort.

Now, people sometimes think that when we try to create images in our minds they should be like photos – clear and sharp. In fact, they don't have to be anything like that. Sometimes imagery only gives us a 'sense' of something, and we never see anything clearly. So, imagery doesn't have to mean fully formed pictures – very often it consists of just fleeting impressions.

People often say they're not particularly visual or good with fantasy. But supposing I say to you the word 'bicycle'. What popped into your head? Now suppose I ask you, 'Where are the brakes on a bicycle?' What pops into your mind now? How does your mind provide you with this information so that you can answer the question? Basically, you're running images in your head – without even trying to.

Now, in working with imagery we're interested in the way certain images are related to certain feelings and mental states. So, for example, if you have an interview coming up tomorrow and are worried about it, you might have images and thoughts popping into your head that make you anxious. However, you might take your children to the park and find that playing with them distracts you, so that after a while you feel less worried and forget all about tomorrow. But then, after the children have had their tea and are in bed, you're lying in the bath and you suddenly remember the interview. In a flash, the anxious images pop into your mind again (a stern figure behind a desk, a dark room, the feeling of nervous perspiration on your hands) and up comes the anxiety again. Now, if we imagine the interviewers are going to be very supportive, kind and interested in us, that the room is going to be comfortable and pleasant, we might have a different emotional experience. We are likely to feel far less anxiety than if we imagine they're going to be very tough, aggressive and critical. So, the nature of the image will have a major impact on how anxious you feel.

Images that set off our anxiety typically come to us at the end of a hard day, in our dreams, or while we are between sleep and waking. They can even wake us up! But rather than letting those images come and go as they please, we can actually turn this ability to fantasise and imagine to our advantage by deliberately choosing images that will stimulate the soothing system rather than (say) the threat system. One way to do this might be to begin by focusing on the feelings of contentment and safeness in a particular place. We call this 'soothing place' imagery and will explore how to help you do this a little later in this chapter.

Developing your 'soothing place'

Some of us, when we are distressed, naturally conjure up images of being in a better place, maybe somewhere we remember from the past or hope to be in the future. Now, of course, we may do this simply to escape or avoid difficult feelings or situations. However, we can also use this tactic to help us cope with difficult situations without avoiding them, by learning ways of containing and creating soothing feelings within ourselves.

The 'soothing place' exercise encourages feelings of safeness and calmness to help activate our soothing system; and when it is engaged it becomes easier to think about our difficulties from a more compassionate perspective and also to experiment with new ways of coping. Developing a soothing place does not mean that we either accept or ignore bad things happening to us, or that we do not try to change things in our life. It is simply a step towards feeling calm enough to tackle these things without resorting to overeating as a way of coping with difficult feelings that may arise.

It is important to distinguish between safety (feeling safe from harm) and safeness (feeling calm, content, cared for and welcome). If people have experienced a lot of threat, particularly from others, they often imagine a place that protects them (for example, a castle with guard dogs and watchtowers that no one can come into) or a place they can hide in where no one can find them. This is really seeking safety from harm and is important but means we will always need to build bigger walls or have stronger protectors to keep danger out, as our minds will always focus on more extreme ways we are at risk unless we address our threat system in the real world. Safeness is a physical and psychological state associated with soothing, where we feel calm, content and able to rest, and is a step towards connecting with ourselves or others. This is the system we have been trying to develop in this section. That does not mean that being safe from harm is not important, and we often need to do this before we can develop our soothing system.

You can use Worksheet 2 on page 144 to help you create your image. I suggest that you work out what you think will be soothing for you on paper before you try to imagine it. This has a number of advantages: it will give your mind time to explore options before committing to a specific image, and it can help you review the image you have chosen to make sure that it does not have any baggage that will move you out of soothing (for example, building it on a memory of a place in the country you used to find soothing in real life but which has now been turned into a housing estate!). I suggest you read though the next section, jot down any ideas you have and then fill in the worksheet at the end. Your soothing place is not fixed in tablets of stone, and you can change it whenever you want. Some people like to create multiple soothing places, so they can choose what feels right for them on the day. Indeed, your brain may flit between images. This is perfectly normal – it is doing the job you gave it, to find imagery that will help you feel soothed and give you choices for how to do this.

Some people have clear ideas about places they like or feel soothed in, but others don't. If nowhere springs to mind for you, it's a good idea to try thinking about the sorts of places you could feel soothed in before you do the exercise. So, when you have some space and time to fantasise, ask yourself what sort of a place would make you feel soothed. Would it be outside or inside? If outside, what would the weather be like? What colours would there be around you? Try to engage in the exercise with curiosity and interest, as if you were an artist designing something for the first time, seeing if you like this here or prefer that there.

Some people like to have an actual picture of their soothing place to focus on while they do the exercise. Other people like to have smells or sounds around them that they associate with their soothing place. For example, one person I worked with liked to have a particular hand cream with her. These kinds of associations can be helpful in activating your soothing system in day-to-day life, as you may be able to keep the sound on your smartphone or the smell on a handkerchief, and use them to rapidly activate your memory of safeness at any time where you feel under threat.

Some people find it helpful to see themselves in their soothing place; to imagine the look on their face, and how they would sit or lie when they were feeling soothed. Others prefer just to imagine their place and their feeling of being in it. It is OK to do either. There is no 'right or wrong'. You may find that different images work better at different times of the day, or when you are experiencing different levels or kinds of threat or distress.

After a little practice, you may find an image that really works for you. Remember, it is not going to be in complete 'HD 3D surround sound and smell-o-vision' – it's an internal image, not a high-tech film – so the more reminders you can develop to help you focus on your image, the better. When you have a soothing place you find helpful, you can write your own script to help you recall and stay in it. You might even want to record this to play back to yourself.

Feeling wanted

After you've been in your soothing place for a few minutes and when you're ready, just dwell on the fact that this place is *your* creation, and therefore really welcomes you and wants you to be here. The feeling of being wanted by a place may seem strange but try it and see how you get on. Just focus on feeling that you are in harmony with this place. You might find that if you allow your face to relax into a gentle expression of contentment or compassion, this helps with the experience. At all times remember that nothing is being forced here. You're not trying to make yourself feel safe in this image; you are engaging in a gentle, curious practice to see how a sense of soothing might develop over time and how your image might change along with that sense of safeness.

Don't worry if you find yourself feeling quite sleepy when you do this exercise. This is quite common, and some people even use it to help them sleep. However, the main aim is to activate our soothing system, so that we can think about our difficulties a little more easily than we can when we are caught up in the drive or threat systems.

Worksheet 2: Building your soothing place

Where would you like your soothing place to be: indoors, outdoors?

What things can you see in it?

What sounds (if any) can you hear?

Are there any physical sensations you can feel (for example, warmth, or textures like grass or fur)?

Are there any smells in your soothing place?

Are there any people or animals you would like in your soothing place? (Try not to bring people in if you have painful memories or feelings associated with them – for example, anger or grief.)

Exercise 5.2: Imagining your soothing place

I have found that many people find it easier to develop their soothing place when they have a little practice in using sensory soothing or SRB. So, we will begin this exercise with this. If you find that you can get straight into your soothing place without it, that is absolutely fine.

Begin by finding somewhere comfortable to sit where you will not be disturbed for at least ten minutes. Bring your soothing system online using sensory soothing or SRB. Read through Worksheet 2, or you can use a recording, to remind yourself of the image you want to create.

You can close your eyes if you feel OK with this. If you'd rather not, focus your attention on the image in your mind, or on a reminder of your soothing place (for example, a particular scent or piece of material, or even a photograph). Alternatively, you can focus your attention on your pebble or shell and imagine your soothing place.

When you feel you've got some kind of fleeting, impressionistic idea of a soothing place, you can start trying to fill out the detail by going through your sensory impressions, starting with the visual ones – for example, what sort of colours are around you? If you're outside, are you on a beach (is it sandy, rocky, pebbly?), in a garden (formal or wild, what kinds of flowers or other plants?) or perhaps in the country (are there trees around, animals in the fields, is the sky blue or cloudy, or is the sun rising or setting?)? Then think about any sound you can hear, because sometimes people find sounds create a sense of safeness. One person I worked with liked to imagine the sound of a little waterfall. You might hear birdsong or the crackling of a log fire. Then think of any other sensations, such as a gentle cooling breeze or the warmth of the sun on your face, perhaps the smell of hay or of a salt breeze on the shore. Going through the sensory details of the image can be quite helpful to fix it and make it real. When you feel you have a place that works for you, give yourself permission to feel wanted by your soothing place.

Your wandering mind will take you away from this place. So just notice where it goes, and then gently return your attention to the elements that feel most soothing. When you have the image back, gently expand it again to other parts of your soothing place.

Affiliative soothing

Some people tell me that their soothing tends to rely on things they do on their own or on eating. This is not unusual as sadly not every human we meet will be caring and compassionate, and experience may have taught us to expect the worst from people. If this is the case, you may need to rely on the soothing activities we have discussed in this chapter until you feel ready and able to engage in more supportive relationships. However, human brains evolved to be very sensitive to caring signals from others and to engage in mutually caring relationships. These can quickly activate our soothing system. If you feel able, you may wish to develop connections with people who help you to feel soothed and build them into your daily life more frequently.

My personal reflections on Chapter 5

‹◇◇›

You might find it helpful to write down your key personal learning points from this chapter.

- Which of the exercises in this chapter do you think you could try at least once per day for several minutes?

- Which would you like to try for a little longer every day?

- Which do you think could be helpful when you need to turn on your soothing system, particularly if you have been in your threat system?

- Is there anything that frightens you about turning on your soothing system? If so, please make a note of what worries you as we will return to this later, to see if your compassionate mind can help you address these fears.

- Are there any thoughts that would mean you would be resistant to trying out soothing exercises or practical things blocking you from doing them? Again, please make a note as we will look at how to address these later.

‹◇◇◇›

SUMMARY

In this chapter, we have explored a number of ways to help you develop your abilities to observe your thoughts, feelings and bodily experiences, to focus your attention and to deliberately bring your soothing system online – for the pleasure it can bring, as a way to improve your ability to manage and recover from threat, and as a bridge to your compassion system. In the next chapter we will explore different ways for you to bring your compassionate mind online. At the end of this chapter, I have included an example of a 14-day soothing system challenge (Worksheet 3). Of course, you can do this over as many days or weeks as you wish; however, setting yourself a challenge, and planning how to fit mindfulness and soothing into your life, will help you build the capacity to move on to the next phase of this book – building your compassionate mind and using it to help you with overeating.

When you have completed the challenge, you can use the worksheet to see which exercises work best for you, and if some are better for certain types of threat. Once you feel you can bring your soothing system on, even if it is only for a few seconds, you can use it to prepare your mind for compassion – which I will help you to do in the next chapter.

Worksheet 3: 14-day soothing challenge

Day and activity	Where did I do this, how often, for how long?	My reflections
Example: **Day 1** Mindful attention to my breath. Noticing when I was in my soothing system.	Three times – when I got up, at midday before lunch, and an hour before bedtime. I did the first exercise in my bedroom. I did the others in the living room – three minutes each time. When I was having a bath, when my friend called me.	I found it very difficult to focus on my breath. I found a pebble and found it easier to focus on that. My mind wandered a lot to my worries about overeating yesterday. I liked the warm water but sometimes worried about overeating. My friend's phone call was nice, we had not spoken for a while, and it helped me to feel calm and cared for.
Day 1		
Day 2		
Day 3		
Day 4		

Day 5		
Day 6		
Day 7		
Day 8		
Day 9		
Day 10		
Day 11		
Day 12		
Day 13		
Day 14		

6 Switching on the compassionate mind

In Chapter 4, we explored how different mindsets can affect our motivations, thoughts, feelings and behaviours. In Chapter 10, we will build upon this idea to help you develop a personal understanding of the different mindsets you experience in relation to food and eating. In this chapter we will work on developing your 'compassion mindset' to help you deal with the experiences that in the past have led you to turn to food to help you, and to manage any emotional consequences of giving up overeating.

Later, we will look at how to switch from a dieting or a comfort-seeking mindset to a compassionate one. But first it's worth looking at how switching mindsets occurs naturally. Let's imagine we are walking down the street planning our next diet. We are likely to be thinking about why we want to diet, the food we need to buy, the activities we will start doing to lose weight, and all of the good things that will happen for us when we do so. We may even start to experience some of the positive feelings we associate with being successful in losing weight. At this point our attention is focused inwards, towards our future plans and what we expect to get from dieting. Suddenly we see a small child run out into the road. A car skids to a halt and the child is standing in the middle of the road crying. We will almost certainly find that our attention has instantly switched to the events going on around us. We are focused on the child's distress and rush to help them, perhaps putting an arm round them and helping them to the pavement. We may look around to see if their parent is nearby or, when we feel the child is safe, look after the shocked driver.

Without our making any conscious decision, the event has switched on our compassionate mindset. Our response has been automatic; we haven't decided not to think about our diet any-more, we've just forgotten about it as something more important has claimed our attention. This switch is often associated with a rapid change in our thoughts, feelings and bodily experiences. Witnessing this type of incident can be quite upsetting and we may feel sympathy for the child, parent and driver. We may dwell on how things could have been far worse, or on the things we wanted to do to help but couldn't (for example, stopping the child before they ran into the road). We may feel a bit shaky, even tearful. A little later, once the incident is over, we may find that our compassionate mind focuses on other ways we could have helped, or on wondering how the people involved in the near miss are. Or we may find that another mindset takes over to help us with the distress that the incident has called up in us. We may use our comfort eating mindset to calm us or our dieting mindset to take our thoughts away from what we have witnessed.

If we could stay with our compassionate mind, but redirect it towards ourselves, we could better understand and sympathise with the distress that seeing this incident has caused us. This response is likely to help us manage our feelings better than either the dieting or the comfort eating mindset, and to enable us to react in compassionate ways if we are faced with a similar situation in the future. This response may congratulate us on our humanity, and value our compassion for others, while at the same time thinking about ways in which we can support ourselves while we're still feeling upset about what we've seen – for example, talking it though with someone else. It may focus on the good we *have* done, rather than on all the things that we *could have* done.

As you can see, our minds are pretty flexible, with the ability to refocus to help us to manage life's challenges. And our compassionate minds can switch on automatically for other people. However, we can find it a lot harder when it comes to being compassionate with ourselves.

Exercises to develop the compassionate mind

The exercises in this chapter use our memories and imagination and are designed to create the feelings that accompany the experience and practice of compassion, both towards others and ourselves. They are adapted from those on The Compassionate Mind Foundation's website, with the kind permission of Professor Paul Gilbert and the foundation. Many people that I have worked with find the structure that these exercises offer very helpful. It is important that you work through them at your own pace and decide which work best for you.

The exercises that follow are focused on four areas:

1. *Developing the inner compassionate self.* In these exercises we will be focusing on creating a sense of a compassionate self, just as actors do if they are trying to get into a role.

2. *Compassion flowing out from you to others.* These exercises focus on the feelings in your body when you fill your mind with compassionate feelings for other people.

3. *Compassion flowing into you.* Here you will focus on opening up to compassion, to stimulate areas of your brain that are responsive to the compassion of others.

4. *Self-compassion.* This set of exercises is designed to direct your capacity for compassion towards yourself. This is just as important as changing your eating patterns. Working on the things that can make us overeat can be difficult and learning how to generate self-compassion can be very helpful during these times, particularly to help us with our emotions.

Developing the inner compassionate self

As we have seen, we all have the capacity to experience different mindsets and act accordingly. We are people of many parts! In the following exercises we will be working to develop the compassionate part of ourselves. Remember that the key qualities of the compassionate self we explored in Chapter 4 are wisdom, strength, warmth and responsibility.

It can be helpful to practise focusing on each of these key qualities in turn and imagine having each one, noting what it feels like and any effect this has on your body and mind.

Exercise 6.1: Imagining the compassionate self

This exercise is designed to help you focus on the feelings associated with creating compassion in yourself. It is hard to offer compassion if we don't have a good idea what this feels like. Please keep in mind that it doesn't matter whether you feel you have these qualities or not. It is the act of imagining that you have them that is important. This is the kind of approach that 'method actors' use to get into a role, as it stimulates certain qualities in their minds and bodies, and as a result their acting is convincing, because for the short time when they are 'in character' they in effect 'become' that character. Of course, when they come out of the role, they may not want to be anything like the character (particularly if they are playing someone like Hannibal Lecter!). Whereas in compassion focused work the idea is that over time you will want to retain the aspects of the role you've been practising. For the purposes of this exercise, it's just putting yourself into that mental state that's important. As with so many of the exercises in this book, the more you practise this, the easier you are likely to find it.

What you will do in this exercise is take each of the qualities – wisdom, strength, warmth, responsibility – in turn, hold it in your mind and imagine yourself having it. Work through each quality steadily, playfully and slowly. You may find some easier to imagine yourself having than others – and this is perfectly normal. Try to notice how each quality can affect your body differently. Remember that you may get only glimmers of images and feelings, perhaps because your mind wanders, or you can't really focus. This is very typical of what happens when we're trying something new, just as if we were learning to play the piano – we'd be all fingers and thumbs to start with, but regular practice will help us improve.

Find a place where you can sit quietly and will not be disturbed for at least ten minutes. Bring your soothing system online using any of the exercises from the previous chapter that you found helpful. When you feel that your body has slowed down (even slightly), you are ready to practise imagining that you are a very deeply compassionate person. Think of all the qualities that you would ideally have as that compassionate person. Try to spend at least one minute focusing on each quality – longer if you can.

Now focus on your desire to become a compassionate person and to be able to think, act and feel compassionately. Imagine having a wisdom that comes from your understanding about the nature of our lives, minds and bodies. You are wise enough to know that much of what goes on inside of us is not our fault but the result of our evolution and of experiences over which we had no control.

When you have a sense of your wisdom, you can switch to imagining having strength. Explore your body posture (sitting or standing assertively) and your facial expressions when you are in this mode. Keep your head upright rather than letting it drop forward; your posture should be one of confidence. Remember, you are imagining yourself as a person that understands your own difficulties and those of others in a non-judgemental way, and who has the confidence to be sensitive to suffering and to tolerate distress in order to gain better understanding of how to alleviate it.

When you have a sense of your wisdom and strength, you can switch to focusing on qualities of warmth – a gentle friendliness. Imagine being warm and caring. Create a compassionate facial expression. Try to imagine yourself speaking to someone and hear the warm tone of your voice. Now reach out with that warmth to feel what it might be like to offer it to another person or animal.

Next, switch to imagining feelings of responsibility. Imagine that you have lost interest in condemning or blaming and just want to do the best you can to help yourself, and others, move forward. Hold on to your compassionate facial expression and warmth but focus now on this experience of committing yourself to a compassionate path of self-development.

Finally, you can imagine yourself having all of these qualities and incorporating them into the way you are with yourself and others.

When you have finished, bring yourself gently back into the room. You might want to write down what it felt like to have these qualities and how it might affect the way you want to act in the future.

Exercise 6.2: Me at my best

Another way you can explore and get close to the idea of your compassionate self is to remind yourself of a time when you felt compassion or acted in a compassionate way – it doesn't matter to what degree. When we are struggling with difficult things in our lives it can be easy to forget that we have the capacity for compassion at all, so actively bringing these memories to mind can help you to remember that you do have these qualities within you and to bring them to the fore again. You can think of your compassionate self as 'me at my best'.

When you have decided on the memory you want to use, it can be helpful to begin by bringing your soothing system online. Then bring to mind a time when you were compassionate to somebody and were satisfied with how helpful you were. Try not to focus on times when you have been compassionate with someone who is very distressed – especially if this is the first time you've tried this exercise. It may help to write down the specific memory you want to focus on, and to 'risk assess' it first, making sure it is not too distressing for you to work with, otherwise you might find yourself focusing on the other person's distress, and maybe your inability to alleviate it entirely. The aim is to focus on your feelings of wanting to help and capacity for compassion.

Once you have brought to mind an appropriate occasion, focus on your body position, facial expression and tone of voice as you offered your wisdom, strength, warmth and courage. Spend sufficient time on this exercise to really be able to explore it thoroughly and reflect on the experience.

Exercises 5.1 and 5.2 both draw on Buddhist ideas to do with developing key qualities of the self (such as mindfulness and compassion), which in turn give us new insights into the nature of who we are and can be. When we see the compassionate self as the self we would like to become, this is no different from wanting to develop any other aspect of ourselves. If we want to be good at sport, an accomplished pianist, a good cook or well-read in poetry – we know that the more we practise, the closer we get to being what we want to become. Some days our practice won't go very well, but this doesn't mean that, over the long term, we can't move towards our goal. It's exactly the same with the compassionate self. We can make a decision to become more like the compassionate self of our imagination. We can practise what we would like to become by imagining, enacting, thinking and playing with those compassionate qualities. If we have an argument with somebody, we can reflect on how we might deal with that situation better in the future. If we have problems with food, we can learn to be compassionate, rather than angry and critical about the way we eat, and think about how to help ourselves next time. There is nothing fixed about our personality – we can make choices about it, and with practice can move closer to the kind of person we want to be. You might find Worksheet 4 to be a helpful way to organise your thoughts and help you keep your focus when practising.

Worksheet 4: Me at my best

The memory I want to use for when I am compassionate is:
What did I pay attention to while I was being compassionate?
What did I feel in my body and what was I motivated to do while I was being compassionate?
What body posture and facial expression did I have?
What was my tone of voice?
What would life be like if I could be this version of myself more often?

Compassion every day

Ideally, try to practise 'becoming a more compassionate self' each day. You can fit practice into even the smallest slots in a busy life. When you wake up in the morning, try to spend a few minutes practising. As you lie in bed, bring a compassionate expression to your face, and focus on your real desire to be wise and compassionate. Remember, inside you, you have the capacity for wisdom and strength – but you have to create space for it. If you practise for even two minutes a day, every day, it is likely to have an effect. You may then find you'll want to practise for longer periods and to make more time during your day for this. Furthermore, whenever you are aware of the opportunity, even sitting in a meeting, you can use soothing exercises to focus on becoming the wise, compassionate, calm, mature self you want to be.

The flows of compassion

Compassion is a three-way street, crucial for our wellbeing; it helps us to deal with threats and challenges and to flourish and grow. In the sections that follow, we will explore these three flows: being able to experience compassion from others, towards others and for ourselves. It is sometimes easier to allow ourselves to be compassionate to others (animals, people or nature) than to allow others to be compassionate towards us, or to offer compassion to ourselves. So, we will start with that.

Compassion flowing out from you to others

The idea of the next three exercises is to focus on the desire to help and on feelings of caring and warmth. If these don't come easily, don't worry; it is your behaviour and intentions that are important – the feelings may follow on behind. In Exercise 6.3 we simply get into our compassionate mindset and imagine our compassion flowing into someone we care about, giving them three key compassionate messages. In Exercise 6.4, you will be focusing on helping a person you care about who is struggling with something in their life and who you would like to support using your compassionate self.

The final exercise in this group (Exercise 6.5) can be a little trickier. Many people who overeat are actually critical of others who overeat and find it difficult to be compassionate with them, as we can be very critical of what we see in the mirror! One way to overcome this is to personalise things; it can be far harder to be uncompassionate with a specific person than with an idea or abstract group of people. Exercise 6.5 builds on your innate wisdom and compassion for others by directly focusing your attention on offering compassion to people who overeat.

Of course, many people who overeat are very sympathetic to the struggles of others but find it difficult to offer themselves the same level of compassion. Indeed, I find this all the time in the groups I run. Exercise 6.7, later in the chapter, is the beginning of offering yourself compassion – but please only try to work on it when you feel that you can do exercises 6.3 and 6.4 quite comfortably and are starting to feel your compassionate qualities coming online – even if only a little.

Exercise 6.3: Focusing compassion on others

First, find a time and place when you can sit quietly without being disturbed for at least ten minutes. Now try to create a sense of being a compassionate person as best you can. Some days this will be easier than others – even just the slightest glimmer can be a start. Now bring to mind someone you care about. This might be a friend, parent, child or pet. When you have this individual in mind, focus on directing towards them three basic thoughts (if you're familiar with Buddhism, you may recognise this traditional text or mantra):

May you be well.

May you be happy.

May you be free of suffering.

Keep in mind that it is your behaviour and intentions that are important – the feelings may follow on behind. Be gentle, take your time, and allow yourself to focus on desires and wishes you create in yourself for the other person or animal. Maybe picture them smiling or looking affectionately at you and being happy to receive your compassionate wishes. Spend time focusing on this genuine desire of yours for the wellbeing of another individual.

If your mind wanders, just gently bring it back to the task. Try to notice any physical sensations or emotions that emerge from this exercise. Don't worry if nothing much happens at a conscious level; the act of having a go is the important thing. It's like getting fit – it may take several visits to the gym or training sessions before you consciously notice feeling different, but your body will be responding straight away.

Exercise 6.4: Compassion flowing out to others in difficulty

In this exercise we are again going to imagine compassion flowing out from you to another person or animal, but in this case that other individual will be facing a difficulty that you want to help them with. As with Exercise 6.3, try not to choose a time when they were very distressed, because then you are likely to focus on the severity of their suffering, and possibly your inability to dispel it, rather than on your own compassionate feelings. It can help to prepare by jotting down the name of the person or animal you want to help, and the difficulty you want to help them with.

Begin by bringing your soothing system online. Now work through the following sequence, trying to spend at least one minute on each element.

- When you feel ready, recall a time when you felt compassionate towards the person or animal you have in mind.

- Imagine yourself expanding, as if you are becoming calmer, wiser, stronger and better able to help. Pay attention to your body as you remember your feelings of compassion.

- Now imagine warmth spreading within your body and flowing over the other person or animal. Feel your genuine desire for them to be free of suffering and to flourish.

- Now focus on your tone of voice and the kinds of things you would want to say or do to help them.

- Next think about your pleasure in being able to be compassionate.

- To finish, focus on combining all of these qualities in your compassionate self, and imagine them flowing into the other person or animal: your desire to be helpful, feelings of expansion, the sense of warmth, your tone of voice, the wisdom in your voice and in your behaviour.

When you have finished the exercise, you might want to make some notes about how doing it made you feel. Sometimes you might want to talk to the person you have focused your compassion on; this is great if you think they are able to receive and use your compassion. However, the point of this exercise is simply to learn to experience developing the flow of compassion to others in a deliberate and safe way. You are ready to start doing this in the real world when you feel you have the wisdom to know who you can offer compassion to, how it will be received and how to deal with times when it is not appreciated (at least at the time you initially offer it).

Exercise 6.5: Compassion for people who overeat

There are several ways to do this exercise. The first step is to identify the person or people that you want your compassion to flow towards. Some find it easier to offer compassion to someone they know personally who overeats. Other people find it easier with someone they don't know personally (for example, someone from a TV dieting programme, or seen in a newspaper). Other people find it easier to offer it to everyone who struggles with overeating. For the purposes of the exercise, it really doesn't matter which you choose. The key point is to learn to feel compassion for people who struggle with overeating.

Find a place to sit comfortably and bring your soothing system online. When you feel ready, imagine becoming a compassionate person – you at your best. Remember to keep a confident posture and an upright stance. Go through the key qualities of compassion as a secure and wise person, believing yourself to be strong, confident and deeply committed to being helpful. You realise how difficult life is because of the brain that we have evolved with and the life experiences we have had.

Now, in your mind's eye, see somebody who overeats. Watch them. Try to understand that their motives and desires are complex and often distressing. You may also focus on the unintended consequences that overeating can have for them. Using your wisdom, recognise how they're caught up in a pattern of feelings and behaviour that they didn't design and probably don't want. You're not trying to change anything about them at this point – just learning to be compassionate for them and to them. Imagine them getting as much compassion as they need. For example, you may see yourself alongside them saying, 'You're going through a tough time at the moment', 'I can see how hard this is for you' or 'I can see that food is a real comfort for you', or trying to help them find ways to address the problems that cause them to overeat.

Give yourself plenty of time to simply keep your compassionate mind gently focused on what you're seeing in front of you. As you do this, you may begin to have feelings about what would be helpful to the person you're watching. However, if you feel your mind becoming angry, critical or irritated with them, pull back and bring your soothing system back online until you notice these feelings ease a little; then re-engage with your compassionate mind before recommencing the exercise. It is not unusual to have only fleeting feelings of compassion for people who overeat, and you may need to gently redirect several times during the exercise.

When you have finished, bring yourself gently back into the room, and note down how you feel now, and how you might act differently towards people who overeat from a more compassionate perspective. You might also want to reflect on your own experience. What came up for you? Was there anything that surprised you? What would you like to work on to improve your capacity to respond to overeating with compassion?

Compassion flowing into you

Although many of us can see how being offered, and being able to accept, compassion can be helpful for other people, we can find it quite difficult to accept for ourselves. In the next two exercises we will practise allowing compassion from others into our lives. Exercise 6.6 is focused on helping us to remember times when other people have offered us compassion. When we are distressed, our threat system naturally focuses on things that are dangerous to us, and this may mean that we temporarily forget that some people in the world have been compassionate to us. The key here is to nurture those memories and use them as a basis for helping us to engage with those in our lives who can be compassionate, to recognise compassion when it is offered and to use it to help us.

Sadly, sometimes people cannot remember other people being particularly compassionate towards them. This can be for a variety of reasons. Perhaps they are so distressed that it is hard to bring back any memory of compassion from others; or maybe they have just not had many of those experiences. Sometimes the compassion they were offered was conditional, with a price tag that they don't want to remember. For example, they might have been offered compassion at one moment and hostility the next from someone very unpredictable. Sometimes memories of compassion from another are too painful to bring to mind because the person is no longer around, and feelings of loneliness or grief can overwhelm us.

So, it's not always easy to find a memory of being offered compassion. If your experiences make this difficult for you, that's sad, but it's not something you can blame yourself for, nor is it a sign of any failure or personal inadequacy on your part. It is simply the way it is! It does, however, create a practical problem, as you will need to build up from scratch an image of compassion flowing into you from others. Exercise 6.7 is designed to address this need by developing an image of someone or something that can offer us compassion throughout our lives, a compassionate companion we can always rely on. It is possible to do this, even if you have limited experience of compassion from others, by drawing on your innate wisdom about compassion that you used in exercises 6.1 and 6.2.

Exercise 6.6: Compassion flowing into you – using your memories

This exercise asks you to recall a memory of someone being compassionate towards you. This memory shouldn't be of a time when you were very distressed because you will then focus on the distress rather than the compassion: the point of the exercise is to focus on the desire of another person to help you. Try to spend a minute or so on each phase. It is important to bring to mind someone who you think is motivated by compassion and wants to be helpful to you, not someone who was out to exploit you in some way or who expected things in return. Try to choose someone that you don't have current difficulties with or are worried about. You might want to write down the memory before you do the exercise, to check it for 'baggage' (such as grief, anger, disappointment, sadness or other powerful emotions).

To begin, bring your soothing system online for a minute or so until you can feel your body and mind slowing down. When you feel ready, bring to mind a memory of a time when someone was compassionate to you.

- Allow your face to relax into a compassionate expression and your body to adopt a posture that gives you a warm glow or feeling of gratitude as you recall the memory.

- Explore the facial expressions and body position of the person who was caring towards you. Sometimes it helps if you see them moving towards you, or see their face breaking into a smile, or their head tilted to one side.

- Now focus on the important sensory qualities of your memory. Spend just one minute on the kinds of things this person said and the tone of their voice. Then focus on the emotion in the person, what they really felt for you at that moment.

- Now focus on the whole experience, maybe whether they held you, touched you, offered you a tissue or helped you in other ways. Notice how they created a feeling of being soothed and connected in you, and your sense of gratitude and pleasure at being helped. Allow the experience of soothing, connectedness, gratitude and joy in being helped to grow. Remember to keep your facial expression as compassionate as you can.

When you are ready, gently let the memory fade, come out of the exercise and make some notes on how you felt. You may notice that bringing these memories to mind has created feelings inside you, even if they are just glimmers. What came up for you? Was there anything that surprised you? What would you like to work on to improve your capacity to receive compassion from others?

Creating your compassionate companion

Sometimes it can be very difficult to recall memories of people being compassionate towards us, or of us being compassionate. In this case, we can use the wonderful human capacity for imagination to help us. As we found in Chapter 5 when we worked on developing a soothing image, this can lead to profound changes in our emotions and physical feelings. This next section uses your imagination to help you develop your compassionate mind and ability to give and receive compassion, including to yourself.

When we feel and sense that another mind is focused on us with benevolence, it can have quite a powerful impact. Our brains have evolved to be very responsive to receiving compassion from others. We use exercises that will help trigger those responses, because in doing so we create a sense of being soothed and an inner security. So how do we do this if we can't recall any real experiences of receiving compassion? We can practise creating an idea of a 'compassionate companion'. Some people say, 'Well, it's all very well imagining compassionate others, but I want real ones in my life.' Of course, we all want compassionate relationships with other people. These exercises are not meant to replace those. They are designed to stimulate your brain to help you with your feelings and emotions. Developing these aspects of our brain can also help us to feel safe enough to create and foster real relationships with other people. So, it is not a matter of either/or. If I can use a sporting analogy again, practising in the gym is not the same as playing the real game, but it can help us when we do play for real.

Exercise 6.7: Creating a 'compassionate companion'

In this exercise you are going to create your compassionate companion. If you could imagine a being that would encapsulate everything you could possibly need from someone totally focused on your welfare, what kind of qualities would they have? Of course, you are not limited to one companion, you can have a whole bunch of them that represent different compassionate qualities (for example, one to go to when you need courage and another to offer you comfort). It can be human, an animal, a tree, an inanimate object (such as a mountain) or even a colour. Please be careful when you choose your compassionate companion if you are using a real person; be sure that this does not come with any other powerful emotional 'baggage'.

Some people may dismiss this idea straight away with thoughts like 'I don't deserve that' or 'If anybody got really close to me and knew me from the inside, they wouldn't like me.' However, for the purposes of this exercise this is all beside the point, which is *to imagine* that you are the recipient of complete compassion from another mind without judgement in the present moment.

Whatever image comes to mind; it is *your* creation and personal ideal of who or what you would most like to care for and about you. Some people prefer their image to be a colour, tree, animal or a fantasy character. Some can bring to mind a fictional character from a book or film (e.g. Gandalf from *The Lord of the Rings*), while others prefer to invent their own person or creature. You can choose someone you actually know, although in my experience this can be a little tricky. Most people we know are not compassionate all the time – after all, they are only human, like us! It is very tempting to choose someone who has been very caring but may no longer be with us – perhaps a teacher, friend or relative who may have passed away or moved on and whom we no longer see. This image can get mixed up with feelings of grief and longing, which can distract us. If there is a person (or people) you feel you can use without emotional complications (for example, people you used in the previous exercise) this is absolutely fine. You can use them completely or take aspects from them to build your companion.

Whatever your companion looks like, it is important that you give them certain key qualities:

- a deep commitment to you – a desire to help you cope with and relieve your suffering and take joy in your happiness

- strength of mind that is not overwhelmed by your pain or distress, but remains present, enduring it with you

- wisdom that has been gained through experience and truly understands the struggles you go through in life

- a warmth that conveys gentleness, caring and openness

- an acceptance that is never judgemental or critical but understands your struggles and accepts you as you are, while also being deeply committed to helping and supporting you.

You can use Worksheet 5 to help you with this exercise. The key is to focus on the feelings, and on the experience of imagining another mind that fervently wants you to flourish. When you have completed the worksheet, you are ready to begin the imagery part of the exercise.

Worksheet 5: Building your compassionate companion

How would you like your compassionate image to look/appear?

Is it a colour, an object (rock, tree, etc.), an animal, a human? If so, you may want to keep a photo or create a collage, painting or sculpture to remind you of them during imagery work.

Would you like one companion or a group of companions who are good at different aspects of compassion and can show up when needed?

What would you like your compassionate companion(s) to sound like?

Does it have an accent, a gendered voice, a particular voice tone (firm, humorous, gentle, etc.)?

What other sensory qualities can you give to it (e.g. its smell or textures)?

You can use these to remind you of your companion.

How would you like your ideal caring, compassionate image to relate to you?

Will it talk out loud to you or be a voice in your head?

Will it be with you in person? If so, is it next to you, in front of you so you can see it, or sitting behind you, maybe at your shoulder to offer its wisdom and courage?

Will it text you, send you an email or a letter to offer you its compassion?

Will it hold/hug you or keep its distance but gently let you know it is there?

How would like to relate to your ideal caring, compassionate image?

Do you want to accept its compassion, even if this is hard?

Do you want to sit with it, be helped by it or keep it at a distance you feel comfortable with?

Do you want to accept everything it says or does?

Do you want to have a conversation with it to explore the compassion it offers you?

Do you want it to offer you compassion and then decide later how you will use it?

Sitting in a place where you won't be disturbed, establish your soothing system and allow your face to relax into a compassionate expression. Then bring to mind your soothing place. This may now be the place where you wish to create and meet your companion(s), or you can choose to meet them in another place. The key thing is to create the feelings of being soothed before you meet them.

Now imagine your compassionate companion appearing in your soothing place; they may be materialising from the mist, walking in through a door, or appearing in some other way. Imagine them sitting or standing beside you. You may want to touch them or be held by them, and that's OK, but only allow them to be with you in a way you feel comfortable with, and that helps you to feel soothed and cared for.

To begin with, simply practise experiencing what it is like to focus on the feeling that another mind really values you and cares about you unconditionally. Now focus on your compassionate companion, imagine they are looking at you with great warmth and they have the following message for you, communicated in a way that you will hear and accept:

May you be well.

May you be happy.

May you be free of suffering.

Try to allow yourself to open up to the experiences of compassion, in the knowledge that you can always rely on your companion to offer you their commitment to you, their strength, wisdom and acceptance.

You may notice that your mind wanders, perhaps to memories of times when people have not been compassionate towards you. This is perfectly normal. Just gently bring your mind back to the task in hand.

Try to do this exercise for a few minutes, then gently bring yourself back into the here and now and jot down in your notebook what you felt while you were doing it.

Exercise 6.8: Using your compassionate companion to help you

Find a time and place when you can sit quietly without being disturbed. Choose something for your compassionate companion to help you with that has been a small struggle this week. Try not to choose something that is overwhelming or where there are major life decisions to be made. Now activate your soothing system and allow your face to relax into its compassionate expression. Then bring to mind the soothing place where you want to meet your companion. At this point you are ready to begin the exercise. Try to spend at least one minute on each element.

- First, imagine spending some time with your companion and experiencing their compassion flowing over and around you. You may want to touch them or be held by them; this is fine but remember only to allow them to be with you in a way you feel comfortable with and that helps you to feel soothed and cared for.

- Next, focus on your compassionate companion looking at you with great warmth. Imagine that they have the following wishes and hopes for you:

May you be well.

May you be happy.

May you be free of suffering.

- Allow yourself to sit with and open up to these experiences of compassion, in the knowledge that you can always rely on your compassionate companion to offer you their commitment to you, and their strength, wisdom and acceptance.

- Next, imagine telling your compassionate companion about a particular struggle that you are having. Imagine their facial expression and body posture as they listen to you with concern and acceptance.

- If you can, imagine what they would say to you to help you face your difficulty. Perhaps they will come up with other ways to see things or suggest other ways to help you. It doesn't really matter – what is important is that you experience their warmth, strength and wisdom, and that you feel you can express the worries or feelings that are troubling you without being judged or criticised.

- Draw the exercise to a close by once more experiencing the compassion flowing from your companion into you. Allow yourself to take pleasure in the feelings of safeness, comfort and connectedness for a while before you gently bring yourself back into the room.

You may want to note down how you felt about this experience, and any new understandings or ways of coping that you have learned from your companion.

Struggling with the idea of a compassionate companion

It is common for people to struggle to develop this image of a compassionate companion. For example, you might have thought, 'Yes, but this is not real, I want somebody real to care for me.' That is very understandable. It's even possible that doing this exercise could make you feel sad, because we all have an innate desire for genuine connections. Of course, it is desirable to find people who care for us, and to be able to accept their compassion. But, sometimes, although we have these people in our lives, we can't allow their compassion in because we haven't learned how to accept it. Perhaps we can accept compassion but just don't have such people available to us when we need them. Sometimes the experience of allowing compassion from our companion can encourage us to look for and learn to accept it in the real world, which in turn can help us to engage with compassionate people and communities. Your compassionate companion allows you to practise receiving compassion at a pace and in a way that feels safe for you, and from a source that is available to you whenever you need it.

Self-compassion

This may be the hardest of all the flows of compassion we have introduced so far. Many of us struggle to be compassionate towards ourselves. We will take a closer look at why this is in Chapter 7. You might find that 'me at my best' offers a good way in. Alternatively, this is where your compassionate companion can be really helpful. Imagine them feeling compassion for you relating to a relatively minor difficulty you have experienced, ideally one that is not overwhelmingly distressing, otherwise you might get caught up in the distress. As you become more confident in using your compassionate companion to support you, you can always increase the difficulty of the problems or situations that you bring to them. For now, you are simply going to try to practise directing compassion towards yourself using 'me at my best' and your 'compassionate companion(s)'.

The exercises that follow will help you explore this flow of compassion, discover any fears, blocks or resistances, and work out which is your preferred method for offering yourself compassion. This may well change over time, or according to the issues you are facing – that's perfectly normal and shows your innate wisdom in finding the type of companion you need to help you when you need it.

In the previous exercises you have practised offering compassion to a person, or people, who overeat. You may have found this tricky, particularly if you are very critical of your own eating habits. Offering compassion to yourself for overeating is really important, but probably not the easiest place to begin your journey. Instead, you may want to offer yourself compassion for other difficulties in your life – perhaps the things that trigger your overeating.

Of course, we know that your compassionate companion is not real: it simply represents the strongest, wisest and warmest parts of you. However, it can be a useful bridge until you are able to offer yourself compassion directly. You can try Exercise 6.9 to get you started. It is similar to Exercise 6.4. The only difference is that you are focusing your compassionate attention on yourself, rather than on someone else.

Exercise 6.9: Self-compassion

Find a time and place when you can sit quietly without being disturbed and turn on your soothing system. Now try to create a sense within yourself of being a compassionate person. You can use the 'me at my best' exercise (Exercise 6.2), or your practice of being a compassionate person, to help you. When you can do this, bring to mind a picture of yourself. Sometimes it can help to use a photograph or look at your face in the mirror. If you have a strong sense of self-dislike or self-criticism for the way you are now, it may be helpful to use an image of yourself as a child.

When you have an image in your mind, focus on directing towards yourself the same three basic feelings and thoughts:

May I be well.

May I be happy.

May I be free of suffering.

Keep in mind that it is your behaviour and intentions that are important – the feelings may follow on behind. Maybe you can picture the image of you smiling back at your compassionate self and feeling joy and gratitude.

Try this for a couple of minutes at first, then gradually build up to about ten minutes when you feel ready. Your wandering mind is likely to be very active, particularly at first. This is quite normal; just gently bring it back to the exercise.

When you have finished, note down any thoughts or feelings that emerged while you were doing the exercise, or after you had done it, that you might want to take away from it.

The next exercise is a variation on Exercise 6.4. In this case you are practising offering yourself compassion for a specific dilemma or difficulty in your life. Try to resist the temptation to choose something that is very painful for you at the moment. You can work your way up to this as you grow in confidence.

Exercise 6.10: Using 'me at my best' to help me with a difficulty

In this exercise, we are going to imagine compassion flowing from you towards yourself. It can help to prepare by jotting down the issue you want to work on. You may also want to use the photograph you used for Exercise 6.9 or to look in the mirror as you do the exercise. Try to spend at least one minute on each element.

Begin by engaging your soothing system.

- When you feel ready, bring to mind your compassionate self. Imagine yourself expanding as if you are becoming calmer, wiser, stronger and more able to help.

- Pay attention to your body as you remember your feelings of compassion.

- Now imagine expanding the warmth within your body and imagine it flowing over and around you. Feel your genuine desire for you to be free of suffering and to flourish.

- Now focus on your tone of voice and the kind of things you would want to say or do to help you with the problem you are facing. If it helps, you can imagine having a conversation with yourself.

- Next, think about your pleasure in being able to be compassionate to yourself and to accept your own compassion.

- To finish, focus on combining all these qualities of your compassionate self – the calmness, wisdom, strength and maturity, the warmth and the genuine desire to help – in both voice and behaviour, and imagine them flowing into you.

When you have finished the exercise, you might want to make some notes about how it felt for you, what you have learned and what you want to take away from it.

My personal reflections on Chapter 6

You might find it helpful to write down your key personal learning points from this chapter.

- Which of the exercises in this section do you think you could try at least once per day for several minutes?

- Which would you like to try for a little longer every day?

- Which do you think could be helpful when you are in your threat system?

SUMMARY

The exercises set out in this chapter are designed to help you to develop and foster your capacity for compassion, and to learn to direct your compassionate attention towards yourself and others. You may find that they take some effort at first, or that you do not actually *feel* compassionate, particularly towards yourself, for some time. However, it is crucial that you can at least *act* from a compassionate mindset before you move on to trying to address your overeating. This is why it is important to focus on your intentions and behaviour, and that the feelings can follow on behind. It's quite normal to find genuine feelings of compassion hard to generate, especially if you haven't had much experience of compassion from others, or if you have learned to be self-critical. Eventually, though, these feelings do emerge – usually for other people or things before we experience them towards ourselves. It is also normal for these feelings to come and go, particularly when we are distressed. The key is to continue to practise the exercises to gradually build up the habit, like a 'mental muscle'. As you do so, your brain will gradually change to improve your capacity to give and receive compassion.

It is possible that these exercises may arouse strong feelings or memories. This is not uncommon; the important thing is to accept these with compassion as part of you that may need to be cared for.

In the next chapter we will explore common fears, blocks and resistances to compassion, and how to work with them.

7 Problems with compassion

Fears, blocks and resistances to compassion

Being able to give and receive compassion (including to ourselves) is a basic human need. When we can do this our body and brain functions at its best and we are more able to manage the challenges and tragedies of life. However, as you may have found when doing the exercises in the previous chapter, this is not always as easy as it sounds. We often have fears, blocks and resistances to compassion, and these are sadly very common. I come across these in clinic all the time, and you are also likely to encounter them on your journey. This may not come as a surprise, but the first thing we need to do is be compassionate to our fears, blocks and resistances, not beat ourselves up for having them, or avoid thinking about them!

Do you remember David, whom we met in Chapter 3? He had lost a lot of weight after a period of illness and then had got stuck in a cycle of yo-yo dieting and self-recrimination. His reactions when he began to work on self-compassion were typical of many people. David recognised that dieting had made him feel better about himself, more confident and in control. Looking back at the past, he came to see how his eating habits had changed alongside the events in his life, and this helped him to realise how he had come to rely on overeating to manage some very difficult experiences. However, although he could see the logic of why overeating had helped him, he could not stop criticising himself for his 'weakness' in needing food to comfort him, or for the unintended consequences, such as weight gain. David also found it very difficult to be compassionate with himself over the difficult events in his life. He could see that if they had happened to someone else, he would feel sad for them, angry on their behalf and would want to help them, but he felt nothing for himself. When I expressed my compassion for the difficult experiences he had had, David found this very difficult to accept – he even talked about ending our work together, as he felt he did not deserve and could not cope with other people caring for him.

Fortunately, David was able to explore and overcome his fears, blocks and resistances to compassion using the exercises set out in this chapter. At first, he was not able to *feel* compassion for himself, but he was prepared to have a go at *behaving* compassionately. He found that this helped him to recognise the positive changes in his mood and eating that caring for himself gave him, and he gradually learned to value his capacity for self-compassion.

Just like David, many of us are not used to thinking compassionately about ourselves and find it difficult to accept and use compassion offered by others. There can be many reasons for this. Some are the result of the culture that we live in; others may be related to painful experiences in our past or present. In this chapter, we will explore some of the most common fears, blocks and resistances (FBRs) to allowing ourselves to accept compassion from others, and to offering it to ourselves.

Common FBRs to compassion include:

- confusing compassion with pity

- believing that people who need compassion are weak

- believing that accepting compassion is self-indulgent or selfish

- believing that compassion is a soft option

- believing that compassion means letting your guard down

- believing that compassion lets you or other people off the hook

- believing that compassion means getting rid of feelings (for example, never feeling angry if people upset or hurt you)

- confusing compassion with compulsive caregiving

- confusing compassionate self-correction with self-criticism.

Confusing compassion with pity

Both pity and compassion can activate our feelings of sympathy and a desire to alleviate distress. However, unlike pity, compassion also recognises our own and other people's wisdom, courage and resilience. Compassion starts from a recognition that in our common humanity we can all, at times, struggle to cope with life. Pitying other people, by contrast, tends to be associated with feeling superior to them. Understandably, many people have a strong aversion to being pitied, associating it with being seen as inferior or weak. Compassion combines sympathy with respect. It starts from a position of recognising our common humanity. Compassionate minds know we can all struggle to cope and will need self-compassion and compassion from others to help us deal with the challenges and tragedies of life.

Believing that people who need compassion are weak

Interestingly, we tend not to think in this way when we offer compassion to others. We see them as in a temporary state of suffering, which we may be able to help to relieve. We are more likely to think that we are weak if *we* need compassion. This may be related to the emphasis modern culture places on self-sufficiency, or concerns about what other people will do if we show them any sign of 'weakness'. This is often related to the confusion of compassion with pity.

Believing that accepting compassion is self-indulgent or selfish

When we are compassionate towards others, we tend to put their needs first. Many of us recoil from self-compassion if it involves putting our own needs first, because we have been led to believe that this is wrong. In fact, allowing ourselves to experience compassion from others, or giving it to ourselves, is often an important step in enabling us to be *more* concerned for others. For example, when we are in stuck in a comfort-eating mindset, we can be very single-minded about eating, or when we are stuck in a dieting mindset, we may think about little other than our diet. In both cases, this narrow focus may mean that we unintentionally neglect the needs of others because we are just not aware of them. Opening ourselves to compassion, as we have seen, can also mean that we will be more open to being compassionate with others. Compassion is like putting on our oxygen mask first when there is an emergency in a plane, so we are in a better position to help others.

Believing that compassion is a soft option

Actually, developing our capacity for compassion and using it to help others (or ourselves) is hard work! Self-compassion requires us to develop the courage to address our difficulties, often facing problems that our dieting or comfort eating mindsets have helped us to avoid because we could not cope with them in any other way. It also encourages us to face up to and take responsibility for our actions, including those that hurt ourselves or others. Compassion can also require us to be assertive with others, for example resisting the urge to eat if they offer us food that we don't want to eat.

Believing that compassion means letting your guard down

Compassion does mean being sympathetically moved by, and empathically connected to, our distress and that of others, but it is also linked to wisdom. At times, we may need to 'let our guard down' to allow us to find new ways of caring for ourselves or being cared for. For example, if overeating helps us deal with our suffering, being more open to suffering is likely to leave us feeling more vulnerable, at least for a short time. However, our wisdom can help us decide when conditions are right for us to do this. 'Letting our guard down' is not the same as tolerating other people (or ourselves) being mean or abusive towards us. We can wisely decide who we share our vulnerabilities with, but compassion can also be there to care for us and to protect us from those who wish us harm.

Believing that compassion lets you or other people off the hook

Actually, compassion is the opposite of this. Our compassionate mind helps us to understand why we do what we do, to acknowledge the impact of our actions and to look for other ways to live our lives. Avoiding thinking about our actions (which often happens when we feel scared, angry or ashamed) means that we continue with cycles of behaviour that give us short-term relief, but that can cause problems for us and other people in the long run. For example, if we feel ashamed of overeating, we might try to hide it or deny that it harms us in any way. Sometimes when we do start thinking about this, we can become overwhelmed with shame and then start overeating again to rid ourselves of this very unpleasant and powerful emotion.

Compassion involves being moved by distress but also tolerating it long enough to understand what is going on so we can find ways to deal with our difficulties and take responsibility for ourselves. This can be very hard when we start to eat well, as we can feel sad for all the years lost to overeating, and even guilty about what we have done to our body, our lives and the people we care about. Compassion will give us the courage to face this, the wisdom to understand it and the strength to change.

Compassion does not mean we let others off the hook either. It will help us to understand the impact of their actions on us, give us the courage to hold them to account and look for compassionate resolutions, or the strength to move on from toxic relationships.

Believing that compassion means getting rid of feelings

Compassion can definitely help us with difficult feelings. A key aspect is turning towards them. As Professor Gilbert says, compassion involves us 'turning to face our dark side'. We may need to explore these emotions to help us understand why we overeat. Compassion can also mean accepting that we cannot continue to get positive feelings from food as our only way of feeling good without consequences (for example, always being in our 'food as fun' mindset). Compassion helps us explore our feelings, and to understand that there may be other ways to address or turn them on that are less reliant on food.

Compassion also means that sometimes we will need the courage, wisdom and strength to endure some feelings, such as grief, to allow them to follow their natural course. We will explore 'tolerating emotions' in the next chapter. Avoiding thoughts and feelings actually makes things worse, as they tend to push into our mind more often and more powerfully until we take notice and do something that helps us understand and address them.

Confusing compassion with compulsive care giving

As we have seen, one of the key qualities of a compassionate mind is wisdom. This includes understanding what motivates us to care for others (and ourselves). Sometimes what looks like a compassionate action actually comes from the threat system – for example, if we always do the washing-up at work because we think this is the only way our colleagues will like us. When this happens, we can become angry and resentful, or even burnt out, particularly if our efforts are unappreciated. This is called 'compulsive caregiving'. It does not consider our own needs, or the (often) unconscious bargains or learned behaviours we use to meet the needs of others and avoid rejection. It can also lead us to do things for others that they have not asked for or may not even want us to do. Compassion is about a longer-term motivation to alleviate suffering, including our own. Our compassionate mind will want to explore our motivation to do things for others, recognising our limitations and the need to care for ourselves when we do. Sometimes it will need to face our fears (for example, not doing the washing-up) to see if they are real. If they are, we need to find ways to address this, but often they are the result of our threat system working overtime and are less true than we thought (maybe other people will do the washing-up and everyone will still talk to us, or it could become a shared task with time for a nice chat).

It is also possible to get caught in compulsive caregiving when trying to develop your capacity for self-compassion – for example, doing the exercises in this book because you think you will get into trouble if you don't, or telling yourself off if you find it difficult to make time for developing your compassionate mind. If this happens, it is likely you will see the exercises as a chore at best and, at worst, something else you can beat yourself up about for not doing. It may be difficult to make changes in your schedule. Your compassionate mind will support and encourage you to make time for developing your compassionate mind at a pace you can manage, validate your struggles, and encourage and value the changes you can make.

Confusing compassionate self-correction with self-criticism

As we have seen, there is a natural human tendency to look for explanations about things going wrong in our lives as being related to something we have done or failed to do. This starts as soon as children understand that other people have thoughts and feelings that they can influence (for example, smiling to make a parent happy). At this age, children have a very limited understanding of why people do what they do. So, the first explanation for anything going wrong (for example, their parent being sad) is for the child to believe they did something wrong, and that they can change what they did so that it won't make their parent unhappy again. Of course, the average two-year-old may not know that their parent was upset because they had had a bad day at work! This is the beginning of the natural tendency for humans to become self-critics. We rely on people with a more developed understanding of human minds and the world (our caregivers) to educate us – for example, by telling us why they are upset and letting us know it is not our fault.

Many people believe that self-criticism is the only way to make themselves do things, succeed or be good. For example, they might say, 'If I didn't kick myself, I'd never stop eating.' Or they might believe that unless they are critical and 'keep themselves on their toes', they will be lazy, and so they use self-bullying to drive themselves on. Some people learn this in childhood – for example, if they had parents and teachers who focused more on their errors than on the things they did well and the good things about them. As a result, they became very good at self-criticism and self-punishment, but very poor at seeing their own good points, or not used to rewarding and valuing themselves. It is important to remember that criticism based on shaming is very common in our society. We are likely to experience it at school, but we can see it in our treatment of the mistakes of politicians and celebrities in the media. So even if we don't have direct experience from when we were growing up, there is so much of it around us that it can be hard for us to develop other ways of relating to ourselves.

Of course, there will be times when things we do don't go as we would like them to, and when we want to change what we do for the better. Compassion is certainly not about an 'anything goes' approach. What we are aiming at is a way of correcting ourselves kindly and gently, and an understanding that change is often a difficult and long-term process.

It can be helpful to keep a summary of the differences between shame-based self-criticism or self-attacking and compassion-based self-correction to hand so that you can more easily work out which one you're using when you try to correct yourself. The key differences are summarised in Figure 7.1.

Figure 7.1 Compassionate self–correction versus shame–based self–criticism

Compassionate self-correction is focused on:	Shame-based self-criticism is focused on:
• the desire to improve	• the desire to condemn and punish
• growth and enhancing current capacities	• perceived inadequacies and flaws
• looking forward	• punishing past errors and often looking backwards
• encouragement, support and kindness	• anger, frustration, contempt and disappointment
• building on positives (e.g. seeing what you did well and then considering learning points)	• fear of being found out and hiding perceived faults
• specific areas and qualities of self	• the whole self
• success and improvements	• fear of failure
• increasing the chances of engagement	• increasing the chances of avoidance and withdrawal

Source: Adapted, with permission, from Gilbert, P. (2009) *The Compassionate Mind*. London: Robinson.

You can see that shame-based self-criticism involves the emotions associated with the threat system, such as anger and fear. Letting go of this can help you to learn new ways to manage your feelings and to deal with the urges and desires that cause you to overeat. Compassionate self-correction focuses on and encourages your desire to do your best and to improve.

One of the biggest blocks to self-compassion or letting other people offer us compassion is the fear that without self-criticism we will become lazy, less successful or will lack a moral compass. The idea that self-criticism leads to self-improvement is very common and is often linked to a cultural belief that telling people off makes them a better person. When children are playing sport, you will often see parents shouting whenever they don't perform to the standard of an adult professional athlete. The effect on the children is heartbreaking. They become increasingly fearful of making mistakes, lose the joy of playing and, in the longer term, many give up sport altogether.

The same is true when we criticise ourselves. Over time we become more fearful of making mistakes, demoralised and we want to hide. Our self-critic tells us that the answer to motivating ourselves is to beat ourselves up even more! If we really want to reduce our overeating (or correct other aspects of our behaviour), we stand a better chance of doing so if we get into the habit of using *compassionate self-correction* when things go wrong or when we start to feel frustrated with ourselves. A key aim of this book is to help you develop a different relationship with yourself, one that encourages you, helps you learn from mistakes and supports you when things go wrong.

Compassionate self-correction is based on being mindful, open-hearted and honest about our mistakes, as well as acknowledging our genuine wish to learn from them. No one wakes up in the morning and thinks to themselves, 'Oh, I think I will do my best not to eat well today, just for the hell of it.' Most of us would like to eat well, to avoid mistakes or being out of control with our temper, and so on. Compassionate self-correction recognises this. Self-criticism, on the other hand, deals in fear and anger: it is concerned with punishment for things we have already done. The problem is that we cannot change a single moment of the past; we can only change the future, and beating ourselves up is not the best way of helping ourselves to do better.

Compassionate self-correction is linked to a motivation to improve (to flourish and grow). Our compassionate mind does this by helping us think about the best version of ourselves, in whatever we choose to do, but holds in mind our current skills, emotional state and the life circumstances that impact on this. It recognises our positive qualities and values them. It acknowledges there will be setbacks as we work towards our goals, because of life circumstances or the skills and abilities we currently have. It looks to our strengths, both personally and in the relationships we have, and explores how we could use these to help us change. It is wise enough to see setbacks as opportunities to learn and grow, while at the same time recognising and validating how upsetting and disappointing these can be.

In my work as a therapist, I have seen how transformative this can be in supporting people to change and move away from critical patterns that make them miserable, and ultimately less likely to reach their goals. Contrast this with self-criticism. One way to think about this is like a well-intentioned but not very competent sports coach. They notice every mistake you make and then shout at you or give you a disapproving look. They either never recognise and celebrate your success, or they tell you it only happened *because* their constant criticism motivated you. The coach's main feelings for you are not warmth and caring, but frustration and anger, even contempt. They may want the best for you but do not recognise how upsetting this type of criticism is or see that the more they demoralise you, the less well you perform, and they may even drive you to seek a more compassionate coach or quit the sport altogether. Of course, if you wanted someone you cared for to learn a new skill, you wouldn't send them to this type of coach. Indeed, coaching manuals tend to teach people to be compassionate because this produces more successful athletes and teams – and makes coaching more enjoyable for everyone!

Making the transition from shame-based self-criticism to compassion-based self-correction can be difficult at first, but with practice it will become easier. You may already be turning more readily to compassionate thoughts as a result of developing your soothing system and compassionate mind. It can be really helpful to make a note of these compassionate coping thoughts and actions when they occur, perhaps even keeping the list with you to look at when you are tempted to return to self-criticism. In the next chapter, we will look at how you can develop your practice of compassionate self-correction using techniques such as compassionate thought balancing or letter writing.

Many people find one or more of the FBRs getting in the way of their work on developing self-compassion skills and accepting compassion from others – even others they know they can trust. Of course, some people may simply never have thought that they might be able to use this aspect of their personality to help themselves as well as other people, possibly because they have found other coping strategies (like comfort eating or dieting). If this is the case for you, you may wish to skip the exercises in the rest of this chapter and move straight on to the next one.

One way around these FBRs is to recognise them, note that they are very common, don't beat yourself up for having them, and develop your compassionate mind anyway! Some people think about this as being like physiotherapy. If you had a weak muscle in your leg, perhaps as a result of injury, you wouldn't tell yourself that you don't deserve to have a stronger muscle. However, if you have concerns about using your compassionate mind, it might be a good idea to try exercises 7.1 to 7.3 before you move on. You can also come back to them if you find that FBRs come up when you try to move towards eating well. I suggest you do one exercise at a time, and plan something soothing or distracting to do between them. It may take you a few days to complete them all.

Exercise 7.1: My personal FBRs to experiencing compassion from others

Please list any FBRs that you think might stop you letting people offer you compassion.

Exercise 7.2: My personal FBRs to offering compassion to others

Please list any FBRs that you think might stop you offering compassion to others.

Exercise 7.3: My personal FBRs to developing self-compassion

Please list any FBRs that you think might stop you offering yourself compassion.

Once you have identified any blocks, you can try exercises 7.4 to 7.6 to help you think about how you might manage these from the perspective of your compassionate mind. You can use 'me at my best' or your 'compassionate companion(s)' to help you. As always, bring your soothing system online for a minute or two, then bring your compassionate mind online. Please be wary of our capacity to be self-critical when you are doing the exercise. If you notice this happening, just stop the exercise and re-engage your soothing system and compassionate mind before you continue.

I suggest you do the following exercises one at a time. This can be hard work, so have something soothing or distracting planned for when you finish each one. You can always revisit each of the exercises as you encounter new blocks, or if old ones become more challenging as you work with your threat system and change your relationship with eating.

Exercise 7.4: Coping with FBRs to compassion from others

Please try to list anything you could do or say to help you cope with your FBRs to compassion from others.

Exercise 7.5: Coping with FBRs to offering compassion to others

Please try to list anything you could do or say to help you cope with your FBRs to offering compassion to others.

Exercise 7.6: Coping with FBRs to self-compassion

Please try to list anything you could do or say to help you cope with your FBRs to self-compassion.

The 14-day challenge for developing your compassionate mind

Once you have tried the exercises in chapters 6 and 7, you are ready to start your 14-day challenge to help you enhance your compassionate mind. Worksheet 6 overleaf gives you a space to explore any fears, blocks and resistances, and think about how your compassionate mind can find a way to work with these. (I have included the example opposite, of one day's entry, to help you.) Try to devote some time every day to continuing to develop your soothing system and your compassionate mind, remembering that it can be difficult. Don't let this become a chore or something you bully yourself into. When you have completed the challenge, you can use it to work out what exercises best help you to bring your compassionate mind online, and if different versions of your compassionate mind work better for certain types of problems or emotions.

Worksheet 6: My 14-day challenge for developing my compassionate mind

Day and activity	Where did I do this, how often, for how long?	Did it help me to develop my compassionate mind? Did I experience FBRs to compassion? Did I overcome my FBRs?
Example: **Day 1** Memory of me at my best.	I used my soothing image to calm me at home. I was able to recall a memory of compassionately helping someone else for a few minutes.	I found being soothed helped me focus. I picked a memory of helping someone with an IT task at work. I felt good about this, but then noticed my self-critic turned up and told me I could have taught them better, and that it took time way from my own task (FBR). I was able to remind myself that I did my best and that the short time it took was worth it for the person I helped, and it helped me to feel good about myself (overcame FBR). I refocused on the memory and felt good about being someone who can offer compas-sion to others.

Day and activity	Where did I do this, how often, for how long?	Did it help me to develop my compassionate mind? Did I experience FBRs to compassion? Did I overcome my FBRs?
Day 1		
Day 2		
Day 3		
Day 4		
Day 5		
Day 6		
Day 7		

Day 8		
Day 9		
Day 10		
Day 11		
Day 12		
Day 13		
Day 14		

My personal reflections on Chapter 7

You might find it helpful to write down your key personal learning points from this chapter.

- Are there any blocks to compassion you need to work on?

- What do you think life would be like if you could overcome these blocks?

- Have you found any ways to overcome blocks, even if this was difficult for you?

SUMMARY

This chapter is designed to help you explore common blocks to compassion. Please remember this is all very normal and not something to beat yourself up about. Learning our own blocks can help us to find new ways to develop our capacity for compassion and move away from self-criticism and shame towards compassionate self-correction. This is an important step in helping you to eat well, develop a new relationship with food and your body, and improve your wider mental health. In the next chapter we explore how you can use your compassionate mind to help you do this.

8 Using your compassionate mind

In Chapter 6 we explored ways to work on developing our compassionate mind, and in Chapter 7 we examined blocks to compassion. This chapter builds on that work by exploring how to use our compassionate mind in practical ways to help us cope with difficult emotions and thoughts – especially those related to eating.

Managing distress compassionately

Many people find that they eat more when they are distressed, and that doing this helps them to manage their emotions – anger, pain, sadness, guilt, shame, fear, etc. Eating can indeed offer some respite from our immediate emotional distress; however, the relief is usually short-lived because the underlying issues or causes have not been addressed or resolved. Sometimes, these things resolve themselves, but if we haven't explicitly addressed them, we might not know *how* they have been resolved. So, the chances are that next time we are in distress, we will turn to food again for the same immediate relief rather than tolerating the distressing feelings for long enough to work out where their real origins lie and deal with them once and for all.

You might ask at this point: 'Well, if eating works for me every time, why bother to work out what's going on underneath?' Sadly, these overeating 'solutions' are not cost-free; they can often lead to cycles of distress and potential health problems. An example of how this pattern can get established is shown in Figure 8.1. Of course, it is perfectly understandable that we do our best to manage unpleasant feelings in any way we can, and in this chapter we will explore how overeating, often along with a dieting mindset, has developed to help you do this. It is important to take a compassionate view of these ways of managing distress, not beat ourselves up for having used them. After all, until we have other ways to manage that we can really rely on, we would be very unwise to give up something we know works, even if only temporarily.

Figure 8.1 The vicious circle of distress and overeating

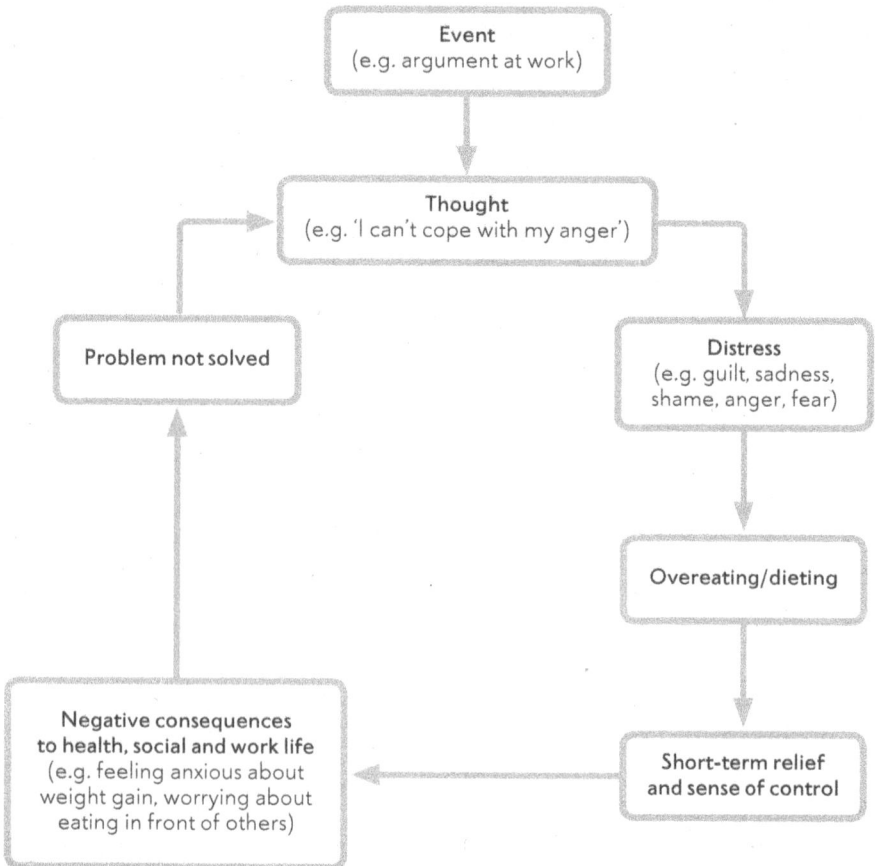

Event
(e.g. argument at work)

Thought
(e.g. 'I can't cope with my anger')

Problem not solved

Distress
(e.g. guilt, sadness, shame, anger, fear)

Overeating/dieting

Negative consequences to health, social and work life (e.g. feeling anxious about weight gain, worrying about eating in front of others)

Short-term relief and sense of control

It is also helpful to remember that, as we saw in chapters 2 and 3, our bodies do respond to overeating in a way that can help us to feel better – and indeed that the food industry has made the most of this fact. So, we're up against both evolution and big business! In exploring alternative ways to manage, we will look at both short-term solutions, for those times when our feelings are very intense, and longer-term solutions, in the form of ways to activate our soothing system and work on our feelings and desires without using food.

Our emotional system for soothing and contentment has evolved to help us manage distress by seeking out and using support from others. When we are very distressed, it can become over-whelmed, and we will use other ways to manage threats. We live in a world that can be very stressful, and where there can be very little space for us to experience soothing – or even acknowledge that we might need it. Indeed, our culture often drives us to associate feeling contented with stimulation: buying new things, eating more food or seeking out new thrills and excitement – buzzes linked to the achievement/drive system in our brain. Sadly, we have lost touch with our need to keep our emotional systems in balance, and the skills of dealing with stress by calming our minds have been sorely neglected.

Imagine your mind as a hot-water boiler. Boilers have a thermostat that switches off the heat when the water is hot enough. Without a thermostat the water just keeps getting hotter and hotter until the boiler explodes. Our emotional regulation systems are a little like this: we have different ways of reducing the pressure. One is 'letting off steam' by distraction, excitement or eating; another is turning our boiler down by using our soothing system.

In Chapter 5, we learned ways to bring our soothing system online so that, in the longer term, our boiler runs at a lower temperature more often! Your 14-day soothing challenge may help you recognise which of these ways work best for you, and if different ones are more effective in helping you lower your emotional temperature at different times, or in different circumstances.

Strategies for coping with a crisis

Practising soothing skills is not a way to stop bad things happening or stop us experiencing the ups and downs of life. No matter how good we have become at self-soothing, we are all bound at some time to experience events, emotions or memories that we find difficult to deal with. We can of course turn to others for support if they are available (remember you made a list of people who can help you on Worksheet 1). If they are not available, or they can't find ways to help us, it is easy to fall back on unhealthy eating, overeating or dieting to get us through, so what we need are other compassion focused ways of riding these waves of difficult emotions and situations. There are basically two ways of doing this: one is to try to *distract* yourself from the emotional distress you are experiencing; the other is to learn to compassionately *tolerate* that distress.

So, let's explore some techniques you can use to help you distract yourself from your distress or to tolerate it, and thus enable you to cope in new ways with the ups and downs and crises of life. It's important to note that these skills are not about resolving the difficulty underlying your distress but are designed to help you to cope with it and to support you while you try to deal with the underlying issue – that is, to give you some space for what may be a longer-term task. These are skills for handling painful events and emotions, accepting life as it is at that moment, when we cannot make things better right away.

In the longer term it is more helpful to learn how to tolerate distress for at least long enough to understand what is causing it, and we explore how you can do this a little later in the chapter. However, this skill can take some time to develop, and even then, we may still want to have confidence in our ability to manage our distress without using food.

Distraction techniques

When we are distressed, or think that distress will overwhelm us, it can help to focus on more positive (or at least less distressing) alternatives. These can include practical as well as mental or emotional distractions. Distractions can also be a great way of 'buying time' to allow our impulses to subside (for example, the impulse to have an extra biscuit as a treat) and help us recognise that we have more control over them than we think.

Practical distractions

These can include hobbies (e.g. knitting, craft work, painting) or sporting activities, going to social or cultural events, calling or visiting a friend, playing computer games, going for a walk, doing paid or voluntary work, reading, doing puzzles, gardening – even housework! It can be helpful to make a list of all the activities you could use as distractions before you need them.

Of course, our minds will still tend to wander, and some things can be more absorbing than others. Some activities, too, have an inbuilt limited time span – for example, a film comes to an end – and we may need to plan a variety so that there is always something else we can do. It can also be very easy to take some distractions to extremes (for example, overworking or exercising excessively). So, it is also important not to let any distraction become too much of a habit, or to get too far drawn into something that we cannot afford to do, because of either the time it takes or the money it costs us. Remember, this is simply a short-term way to help you cope.

Practical activities that help other people can have the double benefit of providing a useful distraction and also helping to activate our compassionate mind. Examples include voluntary work, giving something to or making something nice for another person, or planning and doing a surprising, thoughtful thing for someone that you know they will like. Simple physical sensations can be helpful as a very short-term distraction – for example, holding something cold, squeezing a rubber ball very hard, standing under a warm shower, listening or dancing to very loud music, or singing out loud.

If you have no planned distractions available, or if you are in a place where it is hard to do any of them, you can still practise paying mindful attention to whatever day-to-day activities you're doing: for example, focusing your entire attention on the physical sensations that accompany tasks such as walking to the shops, putting the washing out, doing the dishes, and so on.

Mental distractions

Your soothing place image can also be used to provide a distraction from painful thoughts and feelings. There is also a range of other mental distractions that people have found helpful – for example, imagery exercises that focus on doing something with our distress. Some people imagine their painful emotions draining out of them like water out of a pipe or floating away like a balloon. Others prefer the idea of putting their suffering away but knowing that they can come back to it at a later date – for example, imagining that it is in a box that they can lock away or leave with their compassionate companion.

Another technique is to practise bringing other thoughts to mind so that we give ourselves something else to focus on. These may be positive thoughts about the future (for example, planning our next holiday) or past (for example, happy memories). Alternatively, we can do mental tasks or puzzles, like a difficult chess or Sudoku problem, or a mathematical task – even counting the bricks in a wall takes concentration and so can give temporary respite. Tasks that engage our imagination as well as our rational thoughts, such as following an absorbing book or TV programme, can also help to distract us.

Emotional distractions

Often, we find ourselves so caught up with our emotions that it is very difficult to find a way out of them, or indeed to feel that we have any control over our emotional state. At these times it can be helpful to interrupt these feelings in some way so that we can step outside them to explore compassionate ways to accept and manage them. Again, it can help to plan how you might do this before you get into an intense emotional state, and even to practise learning to switch your moods deliberately to give you a greater sense of control over your feelings. You might want to start by getting into a positive mood, interrupt it for a little while, and then bring it back again. A good way is by using music or TV programmes. Start by listening to or watching something that makes you feel happy – perhaps an upbeat piece of music you really like, or a favourite comedy programme; then switch to something a little sadder – perhaps songs of unrequited love or a tearjerker; then play something that makes you happy again. Notice how your mood can change and how you can choose to allow yourself to go along with this.

You may wish to put together an 'emotional library' of music, films, books, soaps or art that you know can influence your mood. You can use this when you feel stuck with an emotion that you find distressing. It doesn't really matter what mood you use, as long as it is different from the one you are struggling with. For example, if you are feeling angry try not to watch a revenge film; you could watch something that frightens you, makes you cry or laugh, so long as it doesn't exacerbate your feelings of anger!

The key to all of these distraction techniques is to have some available in advance, and to give yourself permission to use them as and when you need them. It can be really helpful to experiment with them when you don't need them. Avoid this when you are feeling really upset. A good way to begin is to draw up a list of possibilities and try to practise a new one every day for a few days, until you find out which ones work best for you.

Exercise 8.1: Developing my distractions menu

Please make a list of the things you have noticed that can help distract you when you are distressed or help you manage impulses to eat.

- Read the examples of practical, mental and emotional distractions in this chapter and add any to your list that you would like to try.

- Pick the ones you think are most likely to work and try them over the next few weeks. Keep a note of which ones work and under what circumstances. For example, doing a crossword puzzle might help you to delay the urge to eat, while listening to music when going for a walk may help manage low mood.

Deciding to tolerate distress

Distress tolerance is a key element of compassion (take a look back at the 'compassion circle' in Figure 4.3. It is also a skill that most of us have to learn. When we are faced by difficult situations, setbacks or disappointments, we are unlikely to think about how much distress we can tolerate: on the contrary, we are more likely to be thinking about how to *stop* feeling bad. So, we will tend to rely on whatever way of doing this we've got used to – and if this is overeating, reaching for the chocolate bar or crisps, then so be it.

One of the things that a compassionate mind can help us with is tolerating some degree of suffering in order to help us gain more control over whether to eat or not when the impulse arises. Now, of course, this isn't simply to prove how much pain we can take! There will be some kinds of distress or discomfort that we can choose to subject ourselves to (for example, giving up unhealthy eating habits) and there will be others (for example, resulting from an argument at work) that we may be able to plan for in advance. In both kinds of situation, our compassionate mind can help us to think about the pros and cons of tolerating the distress (for example, the possible benefits of tolerating the urge to reach for the chocolate bar without giving in to it). By acknowledging our desires in this way, without responding to them, we can learn to act differently in the face of our emotions.

Keep in mind that there can be many different emotions, at a range of different levels of intensity, that might be driving your eating. For example, we can feel angry, fed up, deprived and deserving of food, lonely, or simply wanting to have a good time, and we can feel anything from mild irritation or frustration to utter misery or fury.

If you do decide to practise tolerating distress, be guided by the skills of self-compassion you learned earlier in this book. Don't set impossible goals or see a return to your previous coping strategies as a failure. Your ability to tolerate distress is another 'mental ability' that you may need to develop slowly and to nurture. Here is an exercise that will help you to practise this useful skill.

Exercise 8.2: Learning to tolerate distress

Start with activating your soothing system, then bring your compassionate mind online. Focus on a feeling of genuinely and kindly wanting to help yourself to understand the things that distress you and to allow yourself to experience your emotions. What would your compassionate mind say to help you allow yourself to face and explore your distress without resorting immediately to overeating or dieting?

You might want to include some of the things that people I have worked with have found helpful. For example:

- 'I am suffering these feelings for a reason, so in the future I will have them less often.'

- 'I am able to experience my distress and learn from it.'

- 'My distress will pass; I can learn to ride out the wave.'

- 'I am strong enough to bear my distress.'

- 'This work is part of the long-term changes I can make to turn overeating into a thing of the past.'

Use the space provided below to add anything else your compassionate mind can think of:

Thinking about the disadvantages of *not* tolerating your current distress can also be helpful. For example, you might remember what has happened in the past when you used overeating or dieting to escape the distress of the moment – perhaps feeling cross with yourself and even more distressed after overeating or feeling first elated and then miserable after a diet that didn't last. However, it is also important to remember that at that time you did not have the choices your new skills give you now – don't beat yourself up for having dealt with distress in the best way you could at the time.

From the perspective of your compassionate mind, try to write down in the space provided the downsides of not learning to tolerate your feelings:

Next, try to plan for the types of feelings you want to learn to tolerate, and for how long. To start with, you may want to work on the less painful or distressing feelings that you associate with overeating. Some people begin by working on tolerating the urge to overeat when they are happy or to reward themselves, and to aim at first to resist the urge for about five minutes. You may then decide to go ahead and eat, or to use some of the self-soothing or distraction activities that we explored earlier in this book. The point here is not to stop yourself overeating completely straight away, but to learn at least to *postpone* overeating for a fixed length of time. As you develop your confidence in your ability to tolerate and explore your feelings, you can work on tolerating more painful feelings and doing this for longer periods of time.

The key in this exercise is to use the time that you are tolerating these feelings to be mindful of the things that have caused you to overeat in the first place, perhaps even writing them down. Later in the book we will explore a more structured way of doing this by using a diary (page 245). On some days you will find tolerating your feelings easier than on others; just go at your own pace and use your compassionate mind to guide you.

Compassionate thinking and behaviour

As we discovered in Chapter 4, the compassionate mind has a number of different elements, which we divided into 'attributes' and 'skills' (see Figure 4.3 on page 110). These relate to the way we feel, think and behave. So far, we have been learning to bring our soothing system and compassionate emotions into play, using imagery to focus our compassionate attention on ourselves and others. In this section, we will explore ways to develop our ability to think and act compassionately.

Compassionate thinking

We have seen how the mindset we are in can affect the way we think about things. For example, if we are in a dieting mindset we are more likely to think about the achievements that dieting will bring us, but also all the reasons why we think we need to lose weight, and to be very self-critical if we break our diet. If we are in a compassionate mindset, we are more likely to focus on our discomfort, and to look for ways to alleviate it with wisdom, courage and a genuine motivation to care. The aim of compassionate thinking is to help us stand back from the flow of our thoughts and think in a more balanced way, so that we are not too biased by our feelings and at the mercy of our emotions.

Exercise 8.3: Compassionate thought balancing

One way to develop our capacity for compassionate thinking is to note down the way we think when we are in different mindsets. We can then use our compassionate mind to develop other ways of thinking and express them compassionately. We call this 'compassionate thought balancing'. You might like to give it a try now, using the examples set out in Figure 8.2. First, imagine reading the 'compassionate alternative thoughts' out loud in a very critical or cold voice. Do you think someone would find this helpful? Now read the same thoughts aloud out loud again, this time as if you really wanted to help someone struggling with their overeating. Spend a few minutes thinking about the difference, and how you would feel about being on the receiving end of these things being said to you in the two different ways.

Figure 8.2 Compassionate thought balancing – an example

Overeating thoughts	Compassionate alternative thoughts
There is something wrong with me because I overeat.	*Overeating is very common. People overeat for a whole lot of reasons – because they are hungry, tired, upset or happy. Humans evolved to overeat, so it is normal to have the urge to.*
I am weak because I overeat.	*I don't want to overeat, for lots of reasons, but stopping is pretty tricky. It is a sign of how difficult my brain and body are to manage that I overeat, not a sign that I am weak. It takes a lot of strength and courage to want to work on giving up.*
I will never be able to stop overeating.	*It is sad and frustrating that stopping overeating has been so difficult for me. People can and do learn to change the way they eat and deal with their feelings, but this will take some time. I can give myself the chance to see if the ways of doing it in the book can help me.*

When I lose some weight, I will start to make changes in my life and be happy.	*Losing weight might happen if I stop overeating and dieting, but it is not fair to stop living my life until I lose some weight. I deserve to be happy and as healthy as I can be whatever my weight, and I am going to start doing things to care for myself regardless of my weight!*
If I don't overeat, I can't cope with my feelings.	*It is OK to be worried about this; I have used overeating for years to help me manage my feelings. I can gradually learn to change this, but it is not the end of the world if I do need to overeat from time to time. I will get better at learning to manage my feelings the more I work on it.*
I can't refuse to eat when everyone around me is eating.	*Most people find this hard; after all, eating is a very social thing. But I can choose when I eat – other people around me do choose not to eat at times and I don't think they are bad or rude. I can also choose to eat with them if I want but perhaps eat a bit less than they do.*

Of course, learning to think and talk to yourself in this way, and to believe your new thoughts, is a skill that you may need to practise. You can use Worksheet 7 for this. First write down your overeating or dieting thoughts in the left-hand column. You don't need to develop alternatives straight away. Sometimes we are so caught up in our usual mindsets that it is difficult to think differently. However, if you focus on your compassionate mind or your compassionate self, using the exercises in Chapter 6, you will probably be able then to come back to your list and come up with alternative ways of thinking about these things. You can then practise reading them aloud. Choose the alternatives that you think are most likely to help you, and perhaps keep them with you, either written down on little 'flash cards' in your wallet or purse, or as texts or notes on your phone, so you have them to hand whenever thoughts that are likely to make you think about overeating crop up.

Worksheet 7: Compassionate thought balancing

Overeating thoughts	Compassionate alternative thoughts

Exercise 8.4: Getting outside of your mindset

Another way to develop your compassionate thinking is to explore the ways you normally think when you are in a particular mindset. What kinds of thoughts do you have when you are in a 'dieting' or a 'food as fun' mindset? You can start by jotting these down now. For example, in a dieting mindset you might think, 'I deserve to eat if I am unhappy', 'Dieting will make me feel better about myself', 'Overeating is something I can never resolve', etc. Gently explore these thoughts and see if you can develop compassionate alternatives by using your compassionate mind to try to answer the following questions:

- Is this thinking helpful to me?

- Is this thinking compassionate?

- Would I think like this if I weren't in this mindset?

- Would I teach a child or friend to think like this?

- If not, how would I like to teach them to think about these things? How might I think about this when I am at my compassionate best?

- What would help me in the long run?

The key point is to try to be mindful of your thoughts and to see how they can be pulled in certain ways, depending on how you are feeling. This exercise will help you to stand back a little and observe your thoughts, enabling you to find a compassionate, fair and balanced approach.

Compassionate behaviour

Behaving compassionately is doing helpful, caring or thoughtful things to help ourselves and others to deal with difficulties, setbacks and suffering, and to flourish and improve.

Many people have told me that they have been able to *act* in more compassionate ways before they can routinely *think* in a compassionate way. This takes us back to the comparison with 'method acting' I suggested when introducing the compassionate imagery work in Chapter 6. It's often the case that *doing* things compassionately for ourselves will not necessarily be associated with the *feelings* of self-compassion, at least in the early stages. This is fine – it is our intentions and our behaviours that matter; the feelings can and will come along later.

Learning to behave compassionately towards yourself can help maintain your compassionate motivation. There will, of course, be times when you're angry or frustrated and don't want to carry through on your commitment to looking after yourself with compassion. This is entirely understandable, but if you can, to the best of your ability, just notice and be compassionate to your anger and frustration, and act compassionately towards yourself – it will be easier to pick yourself up and carry on. Sometimes we simply need to ride out the waves of emotion and wait for the intensity to subside.

In the later chapters of this book, we will be working on developing compassionate behaviour in relation to your eating and your body's needs for activity and rest. For now, you might want to try practising acting compassionately towards yourself for perhaps five minutes every day. If you are one of the many people who find it harder to be compassionate to themselves than to others, you might find it easier to do something compassionate for another person, animal or plant for the first week and then gradually add things you do for yourself after that.

Before you try to do this, it can be helpful to put together a list of things that you have done, or seen others do, that you consider to be compassionate. You might also find it helpful to talk to people you know, or to notice what they do, to find out how they are kind to themselves. Here are some ideas to get you started:

- Do one thing, no matter how small, which is specifically designed to be enjoyable (for example, take a warm, scented bath).

- Make time to speak kindly to someone. Try to find out a little bit about them.

- Each day do one spontaneous act of compassion for someone else that doesn't involve food or eating.

- Practise one act of forgiveness to yourself, no matter how small, especially if you tried something and weren't as successful as you wanted to be, or if you had a relapse of some kind.

- Set aside time to practise some of your self-compassion or distress-management exercises.

- Spend five minutes before bedtime remembering compassionate experiences from yourself or other people, that occurred during the day.

Compassionate letter writing

For thousands of years people have found that writing down what they're concerned about can help them 'get it off their chest' and either defuse difficult feelings or put them aside until they are ready to work on them. Writing slows down our thinking in a way that's difficult to do if we just think in our heads. It helps us to become more reflective. Also, we can read back what we have written, and revisiting our thoughts in this way can give us new insights and ideas about what may help us. In this chapter, we are going to focus on composing a letter to ourselves in a style that offers us support, understanding and kindness to help us deal with the challenges of life. We call this approach *compassionate letter writing*.

We can use letter writing to develop our skills in both offering and receiving compassion. Letters can help us to capture thoughts, feelings, new ways of paying attention and new ways of acting. They can also help us to identify blocks to compassion that can occur in imagery work or when we are trying out new ways of behaving compassionately. Compassionate letter writing can be used in addition to the other skills we have worked on in this book. Ideally, as with each new skill we have learned, we don't want to be trying it for the first time when we are in the grip of another powerful mindset that can lead us to overeat. So, initially at least, we will use our letters as a way of planning to manage overeating in the near future. As you become more skilled, you may find that you can use letter writing to help you deal with urges to overeat as they happen, or with other painful emotions or feelings.

We will explore how this can help you put together the information and analysis that you have developed about your overeating, and the skills you have learned so far, in a structured way. Many people have found this very helpful in finding lasting solutions to overeating.

Getting started

There is nothing rushed in compassionate letter writing – just take your time. Having said that, once you are ready and in the right frame of mind, it's useful to start writing regardless of whether or not you know what you're going to write. In fact, in many ways it's a good idea not to work things out too far in advance but to just 'go with the flow'. Sometimes people sit staring at a blank page, going over and over in their heads what to write. This can be linked to the self-critical or judging mindset, trying to work it all out in advance and make sure you do it 'right'. But there is no right or wrong here, and it's fine to start and stop – you might have a number of false starts before you get into the flow.

What 'getting into the flow' really means is allowing your hand rather than your head to do the work, so that you're writing as you think rather than thinking first and then writing. As I say, the biggest block to this is trying to have too much clarity before you start. If you just start writing, regardless of whether what you're putting down seems sensible, or indeed makes much sense, then slowly the flow may come.

There is always the temptation to want to write the 'perfect letter'. I never have, nor will I ever, and nor has anyone I have worked with – but that's OK. What we are looking for is a 'good enough' letter to help bring feelings of compassion to the fore and to get us into the compassionate mindset. So, you may also need to be compassionate with your inability to do 'the perfect' letter whenever you attempt the exercise.

When you feel more comfortable writing letters, it is likely that you will intuitively know what the feelings and challenges are that you want your letter to help you think about and work with. However, many people who overeat can find this difficult to begin with – not least because overeating often helps us manage difficult feelings, and we may be so used to doing this that we're not even aware of precisely what is behind the distress we are trying to soothe by eating. Compassionate letter writing can help you to look at this distress more clearly but also in a way that is manageable, to give you an opportunity to explore your feelings and thoughts. It can enable you to practise bringing your soothing system and compassionate mind together to find new solutions to your difficulties.

Setting the scene for compassionate letter writing

There are several key steps in developing a compassionate letter. Before we even begin to write, it is important that we are in the right frame of mind. To do this you may wish to start by turning on your soothing system for several minutes. Then bring your compassionate mind online.

Try to create a compassionate expression on your face and imagine what your tone of your voice would be if you were to speak. Spend a few moments focusing on what it feels like to be 'you at your best' or stepping into the shoes of your compassionate companion. Remember, you don't have to have a well-defined image in mind, just a presence that you can sense with you, that is focused on your wellbeing and recognises the nature of the difficulty you are struggling with. Imagine the sound of the voice or any communication that comes from them as wise and strong, expressed with great warmth, never judgemental, always understanding and looking for the helpful way forward.

When you can feel your compassionate mind is online, you can begin to work though the various steps to letter writing. Don't feel you have to go right through the process at once; take your time and only go as far as you're comfortable with in one sitting. You will need a bit of time; it's a good idea to put aside an hour or so each time you try it. The key is to feel comfortable with the skills in each step before you move on to the next. You can use your compassionate mind to help you work out if you are ready to move on, and to offer you support and encouragement while you experiment with this new way of working with your thoughts, feelings and eating. You may wish to plan for something soothing or distracting to do after you have finished writing your letter, and to allow yourself time and space before and after your writing session to care for yourself.

Steps to compassionate letter writing

Step 1: Paying compassionate attention to your feelings

This involves either the difficult feelings that you are experiencing now or any you anticipate experiencing in a new situation. Start by bringing to mind the changes in your eating that you want to make, or the situation or feeling that you want to work on that may trigger overeating in the near future. This is likely to bring your threat or drive system into action. Notice how this affects the feelings in your body, and the thoughts and emotions that come up, perhaps making a few notes as you go along. The changes or situation you have in mind will be the focus of your letter, but we don't want to stay with the feelings any longer than we need to work out what our letter is going to help us with. Usually about a minute is enough. It may help to use a timer, so you know when to move away from this phase. As soon as you feel in touch with this, it is time to move on.

Step 2: Stepping outside the feeling

Having noticed with mindful attention the effects that the prospect of changing your eating (or whatever other situation you have in view) have on your threat or drive system, your aim now is to step outside those feelings a little. You can use the soothing exercises you have practised from Chapter 6 to help you. In this way you can experience the emotions that you are struggling with without getting too caught up in them or feeling the need to act on them immediately.

Step 3: Experiencing safeness

If you feel you can tolerate your feelings and move straight into your compassionate mind now, you are free to do so. However, if you are finding it difficult to stay with your feelings – for example, if your threat system becomes too active, or your drive system wants you to do something to change your feeling state – then it can be helpful to spend some time in your soothing system first. When you notice that your threat system or drive system has dampened down a bit, but you are still aware of the feelings that you may need to work with, then it's a good time to move on.

Step 4: Activating your compassionate mind

The next step is to bring your compassionate mind online. This could be 'you at your best' or your compassionate companion. You can do this by working through the process described under 'setting the scene'. It's best not to begin letter writing until you feel confident that you can bring your compassionate mind online, even if only as a fleeting experience.

When we are developing our compassionate mind, we want to make it as much of an emotional, bodily and sensory experience as we can – even if this is only a fleeting sensation. It may also be helpful to have something with you to look at, touch or smell, that helps to keep your soothing system active. When you can feel this compassion, then it is time to begin writing your letter.

The key is to write your letter from the perspective of the compassionate self. It understands, empathises with and supports you unconditionally. It is wise, strong and caring. It will recognise that thinking about doing things differently, or understanding ourselves in new ways, can be painful; so, it won't rush your letter or ask you to make changes that you are not ready for.

It can be difficult to activate our compassionate self, and if you find it tricky, don't worry – this happens to all of us. It may be that this is as far as you can get on your first four or five tries at compassionate letter writing. This is perfectly normal – it can take several weeks, even months, of returning to practise before some people are ready to move on to the next stage.

Step 5: Beginning your letter

As someone who has always struggled to write the first paragraph of anything, I know that compassionate letters can be tricky. I, and many people I have worked with, have found it helpful to follow a structure that gives some idea of where to begin and where to move on to. So, the next steps will set out a suggested sequence of themes. For now, we'll start with a couple of general guidelines.

Recognising your compassionate qualities

In the first part of your letter, it is important to help yourself recognise your own *internal wisdom, courage, strength* and *resilience*. This is because we can often feel overwhelmed by our problem or become locked into a very self-critical way of thinking, and it can be hard to see these qualities in ourselves that we will need to help us face our problems. So, we are aiming at least to remind ourselves that we have these qualities, even if we can't feel them.

First person (I) or second person (you)?

Sometimes we find it hard to write directly about ourselves in the first person (e.g. 'I have been very brave in acknowledging feeling angry this week and in trying to understand why I feel this way'). It can help to write your letter in the second person to begin with, ideally as if it is coming from your compassionate self or companion (e.g. 'You have been very brave . . .').

Imagine for the rest of this chapter that your name is Kwame and that you are writing your first compassionate letter to yourself. You'll start by writing in the second person, beginning 'Dear Kwame', and then go on to recognise the compassionate, wise, brave, strong and resilient things that you feel Kwame has done well over the previous week and in the past. At this point you're not focusing particularly on your achievements but on the qualities of compassion that you want to foster. This part of the letter should also include your own (or your companion's) compassionate feelings for Kwame. For example:

> Dear Kwame, it has been very difficult to watch you struggle with your feelings over the last week and it is not surprising that you have ended up overeating. I understand that life has been hard for you in the past and is hard at the moment. However, I have been impressed by how courageous you have been in trying to tackle these feelings and to understand how your brain and your body work. I have also been impressed by the ways in which you have been able to be caring for others, even though you have been upset, and to carry on with some things at work that you found difficult.

It is really important to try to think about specific examples that our compassionate mind would offer us. You may not even believe it at this point, but it is important to activate that part of your brain that focuses on your compassionate capacities, courage and ability to tolerate and manage distressing things.

Step 6: Empathy and understanding

It is important that our letters allow us to express empathy with and understanding of the struggles that we have experienced in the past, are having now, or may be facing over the coming days or weeks. There are three important elements to this that we will work through in turn.

Recognising that your struggles are understandable

It is really important to understand that the struggles you are having are part of a common human experience. Reflect on what you know about our brains and bodies, your personal history, the situation you find yourself in and the ways in which you have learned to cope with difficult things. For example, you might continue your letter:

> *It is understandable that you would be worried about feeling depressed or anxious this week. In the past people often told you that you weren't capable or good enough, and that is what your body has remembered. When you are struggling, often these memories come to the surface, and you can remember when people put you down and criticised you when you tried to do new things. Of course, you would have learned from this that new things were too difficult to manage, or that your own feelings of inadequacy were the truth, rather than a feeling that was taught to you by other people. It is also understandable that your brain is very good at helping you make these feelings worse, by spending time ruminating about them, pulling in other memories, or thinking about new situations where things might be difficult, and focusing on how you might be rejected if you don't get things right. Your brain is also very good at helping you be sensitive to threats, particularly of being left alone or abandoned, because this is what all animals fear. In the past you found that food often helped you to deal with these painful feelings, or you ate with others to help you to fit in with people you thought would otherwise reject you.*

Sometimes – in fact quite often – you may find it hard to understand why you are struggling with things. You may not recall your history in detail or have a full understanding of why you cope in the way you do. When this happens it can be helpful to focus on what is threatening to you and what your biggest concerns would be if what you feel threatened by were actually to happen now. You can also look at the ways you have coped with these threats in the past. For example, what would worry you about stopping overeating or giving up dieting? We will explore this more in the next chapter.

It is very likely that the threats you have experienced are those faced by all humans at some time in their lives, and your way of coping was the best you could find at the time. You may wish to discuss with someone close to you how you came to cope in these ways. If you don't want to, or there's no one suitable to talk to, it is important to recognise that your ways of coping have helped you, at least in the short term, so it is understandable that you would want to keep them until you had better ways of managing your feelings or difficult situations.

Understanding the unintended consequences of the ways you have coped with threats

We do this not to beat ourselves up for doing things that in fact haven't solved difficulties for us, but to help us recognise some of the costs and pain that these ways of coping have caused us and may cause us in the future. It is a part of recognising our suffering, and motivates us to relieve it in a way that does not involve food. For example, our letter might continue:

It is understandable that you would struggle with feelings of depression and anxiety. It is also understandable that the way you have learned to cope has been to withdraw, to hide away, not to want to share your feelings with anyone in case they hurt you or put you down, and to comfort eat. This has sometimes helped you get through difficult times in the past but might stop you getting the support and care you need from people around you at the moment. It is also understandable that you bully yourself, to remind you to keep yourself safe from other people's attempts at attacking you. One of the unintended consequences of this is that you are now so good at bullying yourself that you end up feeling even more miserable, alone and isolated. It also stops you thinking about other ways of dealing with the things in your life that anybody would find difficult and challenging.

Understanding that it's not your fault, but it is your responsibility

Remember, we didn't ask to be born into the circumstances or relationships we grew up with, and we certainly did not ask to have a 'see-food-and-eat-it' brain, a body that is better at storing food than burning it and a complex emotional system that can easily get out of kilter! However, we have inherited these things and are responsible for managing them in a way that reduces our suffering and lets us take pleasure and joy in the life, body and brains that we have, and frees us to engage in the world around us. So, to continue our letter, we might say:

It's not your fault that you want to run away and hide – this is very normal for any of us when we are feeling under attack or under threat. Nor is it your fault that you didn't have an opportunity to learn that you are capable and can manage life's challenges. You didn't choose to be here, to have your history or to have a brain that is primed for fear and to ruminate on things you are finding difficult.

You also didn't choose a brain that is set up to see food and eat it, or that responds so that food helps you with your feelings. Your over-eating was encouraged when you grew up, by other people and the food industry, and it was the only way you could manage the painful feelings you had then and have now. Of course, you overeat when you're socialising with other people – most people do – but for you this is a way of helping you get closer to other people so you don't feel so afraid that they will not want to be with you.

You do want to find other ways to cope with the threats you experi-ence, and I know you can and will work to find other ways to cope, when you feel afraid, that are better for you.

Step 7: Understanding what you need to help you cope with threats

The next step focuses on understanding what you need to help you cope with your emotions or the situation you are in. This has two elements: what you needed in the past to help you find ways of coping, and what would help you to cope differently now.

What did I need in the past?

For example, you might write:

In the past you needed people to support you, to mentor you, to help you feel confident in managing life's struggles, and to help you find ways of dealing with the challenges that all human beings face. This may have included people to tell you that you were good at things, to teach you how to do things patiently, to tolerate your frustration when you couldn't cope any more, and to support you and help take over some of the things that you found too overwhelming. You may have needed people to be there for you when things were hard and to help remind you that you could deal with things as well. You also needed people not to use food to pacify your feelings.

What do I need to help me cope now?

What we have just written may well be very useful to identify our emotional and practical needs, but sadly we cannot change the past. However, we can change the present and our future by responding to them in a different way. So, we might write:

The first thing to do is to recognise that you are facing difficult challenges at the moment: on top of the ones that every human faces, including dealing with your brain and body, you are also struggling with things at work that are difficult just now. You have too much work to do, and you are worried that people will judge you harshly if you can't do it all.

This is not unrealistic as there is an element of performance-related promotion in your job. However, what you need now are people to understand the amount of pressure that you are under, and to be supportive and sympathetic to that. You need to find ways to manage your workload differently, and perhaps to be more assertive with your managers. Try also to be honest with yourself about the things that make you good at your job, so that you don't feel so threatened when you are struggling. You may need to share some of your worries with people at work who will be sympathetic and able to help you recognise that you are not the only one who's feeling under pressure at the moment.

You may need some support to learn to deal with these difficult feelings and situations without using food. It may help to have a better structure to your eating, and to find other ways to deal with this stress so you are less likely to overeat. You may also need to accept that you will not be able to give up overeating all in one go, and to be gentle with yourself when you eat more than you need to.

Step 8: Developing compassionate coping thoughts and behaviours

The next part of your letter involves considering the ways of thinking and acting that may help you deal with the struggles you face in a different way. Remember that it is OK to allow yourself to keep your old ways of coping until you feel ready to give them up; otherwise, this step can feel like making a list of things we *must* do, and we can then easily fall into the trap of beating ourselves up if we can't do them straight away or if some don't work for us. So, in your compassionate letter you might say:

Everybody struggles with work pressures, and you are no different – remember how often in the past you have recognised that other people struggle at work and have tried to help them cope. Your friends and family may listen to your distress, and it is important that you listen to it too. In fact, several people have commented that you are overworking, and that you could slow down and it would be OK. Perhaps you can look at what work you need to do and what you can schedule differently. Perhaps you can arrange a meeting with your manager to reschedule your workload.

You could also choose to eat with other people, as you know you are more likely to overeat at work when you are alone. Perhaps you could start by having lunch with Raj, so you are a little less hungry when you come home.

Here we can see that a combination of thoughts and actions may be needed to help us cope differently.

It can help to write these down in note form and keep them somewhere that's easy to get to when you want to remind yourself of them. People use various ways of doing this – for example, jotting them down on a flash card, or saving them as a text or voice message on their phone. It can also help to say them to ourselves via our compassionate mind, or even in the mirror, with a compassionate tone of voice.

It may well be that these new ways of coping do not feel at all comfortable, or even believable, at this point. That's absolutely normal. Part of the work you're doing in your letter is to at least identify that there are ways of thinking about and managing threats that are different from the strategies you have learned in the past and used to help you cope.

Step 9: Imagining a compassionate future

When you have developed some compassionate ways of thinking and acting differently to manage threats, it is important to think about how life would be if you could put these into practice. This will help you to explore compassionately the reasons why you might want to think and act differently in the future. One way to do this is to write about what your life would be like if you were able to follow the compassionate wisdom in your letter. For example, you could write:

> *Kwame, I know it's really hard for you to think that you might deal with yourself in a more compassionate way around your mood, worries about work and comfort eating. However, if you were able to, perhaps you wouldn't feel so anxious and fearful that other people*

are thinking critically of you. It might even be that you would feel under less stress at work. You might worry less about what you eat and be able to give up dieting. You might have a better work–life balance. You might even be able enjoy your achievements, be content with the things you can achieve there and tolerate the frustration of the things you can't.

Clearly these are all 'maybes'; however, it is really important that this part of your letter helps you to be open to these new ways thinking or acting. Just play around with them – write down all the possibilities you can think of.

It is likely that you will hear a lot of 'yes, buts' in your head when you are writing this part of your letter. Again, this is normal and to be expected; the key is to notice what the objections are but not to engage with them. If you feel that they are getting in the way, you can pause here and return to focusing on your compassionate mind, knowing that it can help you with these concerns a little later. When you feel ready, you can continue your letter.

Step 10: Making a compassionate commitment to change

In this part of the letter your compassionate self will be supporting you and encouraging you to commit yourself to making some of the changes it suggested in Step 9. The key is to commit to these changes without bullying yourself into making them. Your compassionate self is aware of your limitations, and so you can use it to help you decide what elements of compassionate thinking and action you are prepared to take on right now, and what may feel too difficult to try straight way. It is important to remember that you are moving towards these changes in a compassionate way, and that it is best to do this in small and achievable steps.

You may need to reread Step 9 from the perspective of your compassionate mind ('you at your best' or your compassionate companion) to help identify the things that you feel you can move forward with now. Do remember that it takes courage to try new ways of coping, and wisdom to recognise what is possible for you in the short and then in the longer term. It can help to set out a series of steps that will take you gradually to the point where you can manage your distress in the ways your compassionate mind would want you to. So, for example, you might now write:

> *Kwame, having reread my letter to you, I recognise that perhaps you are not as compassionate with yourself as you want to be, and a bit of you feels that this is your fault too! Perhaps you could try a couple of things to help you be more compassionate with yourself. Try not to blame yourself as much for the difficulties that you have faced at work, and let other people know that you are struggling and that maybe you need their support at this time.*

> *What you could try right now is to phone your best friend Mark, let him know you have had a hard week at work and plan to do something more relaxing together. You could talk to your boss too, but you might need someone to help you do that. Maybe talk to Mark about how you could raise the idea with your boss that work has just got too difficult. You could also ask Raj to have lunch with you a couple of times in the week and perhaps arrange for Danielle to visit you at the weekend, when you tend to be most likely to overeat when you feel down.*

> *You can practise bringing your compassionate mind online to help you feel safer with your own feelings, and work on recognising that they are not your fault. I would like you to be compassionate with yourself all the time, but we both know that this is not possible for any of us.*

I know that you are going to find relaxing very difficult, as you normally feel driven to achieve things. But I would like you to try to do a self-soothing exercise for five minutes a day – though please don't be too hard on yourself if you find this difficult.

Finally, think about how you can finish off your letter. You might do this by summarising the main points, perhaps recognising your courage for reading it, and wishing yourself well. For example, you might draw to a close by writing:

Thank you for taking the time to read this, Kwame. You have faced some difficult decisions while you've been reading this and explored some difficult feelings. This took a lot of courage on your part, and I am proud of you.

Good luck over the coming week. Please remember I will always be here for you if you need me.

Step 11: Paying compassionate attention to your letter

So now you've written your letter – to yourself. The final two steps involve you as the recipient as well as you as the writer. Many people can write a very compassionate letter for someone else, or even for themselves, but cannot 'feel' it; Exercise 8.3 is designed to help with this common difficulty.

Exercise 8.5: Imagining offering compassion to yourself

The aim of this exercise is to help you 'feel' the compassion in your letter, to have the experience of being cared for and supported by another person in a warm, caring, non-judgemental and helpful way.

This is similar to exercises 6.9 and 6.10; here again you are going to imagine compassion flowing from you towards yourself.

When you feel ready, bring your compassionate mind online. Imagine yourself expanding as if you are becoming calmer, wiser, stronger and more mature, and able to help. Now imagine expanding the warmth within your body and it flowing over and around you. Feel your genuine desire for you to be free of suffering and to flourish.

Finding your compassionate voice

It is important to be able to 'hear' your letter in the voice you've used to write it. When we are being compassionate with others it is often the tone of our voice, far more than what we actually say, that conveys our compassion. In just the same way, it's not only what you say in your letter that is important but also the way you say it.

Many people find it really helpful to read their letter out loud and listen to it carefully, as if they were being compassionate with somebody else. It can sometimes help to do this in front of a mirror, or to a photograph of yourself. If you tend to pick on yourself about size and shape, or how or what you eat, it may be better to look at a picture of just your face, rather than your whole body. Often when we are feeling the need for compassion we are taken back to a place in our memory where we feel quite young, scared and unsupported. So, you might find it helpful to read your letter to a younger version of yourself, as we tend naturally to be more compassionate towards children. Even so, many people who are highly self-critical can find this a struggle. Still – give it a go and see what helps you best.

We looked at finding your compassionate voice tone in Chapter 6; you can revisit this now if you are struggling to find this tone.

When you have found a tone that you can use to express compassion to yourself or someone/something you care about, you can try to notice the concern, warmth and wisdom the letter can bring to you when you are in pain and distress, and just doing the best you can to get through life, as we all are.

Now try reading your letter aloud to yourself. Sometimes it can be really helpful to record this and then listen to it from the perspective of yourself when you need compassion. This can make it a little easier to work out which parts of your letter are helpful to you and practise developing an internal voice you can use to support you whenever you need it. If you feel uncomfortable with this, practise reading your letter aloud and notice which parts touch you and help you feel soothed and understood. When you have finished, you can spend some time focusing on the joy of being able to be compassionate to yourself.

Step 12: Enhancing your compassionate letter

As you read or listen to your letter being read aloud to yourself, try to notice your feelings and whether they change when you hear it. Are there parts that are harsh or condemning? This is not at all unusual, particularly in the early stages of learning to be compassionate. If this is the case, you may wish to change these parts of your letter. However, as I said at the beginning of this sequence, it is important not to get caught up in trying to write the 'perfect letter': it only needs to be *good enough* to bring our soothing system into play, and tone down our threat and drive systems enough to allow us to consider other ways of thinking or acting without getting caught up in old coping strategies. No letter you write is ever going to be perfect, no matter how much you practise – and believe me, I have had a fair amount of practice!

Rereading the letter often helps you to see blocks to compassion, and to pinpoint things you can't believe or find hard. It's important to be compassionate with these blocks and to recognise that they are a normal part of the process. You can use them to develop your letter further.

Making time to write your letter

Letter writing can be a very time-consuming process while we are learning. As I said at the beginning of this chapter, you'll probably need to set aside about an hour at a time to practise. You may also find it difficult and frustrating at times. However, it is also empowering to discover that you have this ability and can improve it by practice. It's a skill like any other. We can all learn to play the piano – some of us find it harder than others, some of us take a lot more time to make progress, but it is something we can all become *good enough* at. The key message with compassionate letters is that they don't have to be perfect; they just have to be good enough to:

- help stimulate compassion for yourself, and help you to find other ways of feeling safe with your emotions, rather than being driven to do something about them instantly

- develop new ways of thinking about yourself, and about your shared humanity

- find new ways of coping that fit for you, and that have fewer unintended consequences than your old ones that involved food and eating.

If your letters are putting you in touch with painful feelings, writing them can be quite exhausting, and the feelings may stay around for a little while. It is important to practise compassionate behaviour towards yourself after you have stopped writing.

Try to allow yourself at least half an hour afterwards when you are not doing stressful things. It can also help to have something soothing or distracting planned for when you finish.

Other people reading your letters

Some people find it helpful to share their letters with those they can trust, who are supporting their journey to eating well. This may be family members, friends or therapists. You will need to use your compassionate wisdom to think about whether this will be helpful to you, and if the people reading the letter will be able to understand you and not become overwhelmed or defensive about the things they read. If this is not the case, it can sometimes help if they read the letter to you, or record it for you, particularly if you find it hard to find your own compassionate voice.

Short letters

One way to think about doing a compassionate letter is to liken it to doing long division (something I never really liked!). You can then break things down to shorter coping statements (for example, those used in compassionate thought balancing) or new actions (compassionate behaviour) that gradually become habits. It may be that as your compassionate mind grows, you will develop short letters on paper or in your mind because you know yourself better and can bypass some of the 'working out' parts of the letter. This is absolutely fine; you may only want to write a longer letter for times when you get stuck (for example, by a block to compassion) or have an issue that is getting in the way of eating well and that you don't understand or have a plan for.

At the end of this chapter, I have included a summary of the key steps in compassionate letter writing. You may wish to add writing at least one letter a week to your compassionate practice.

Of course, many people do not like writing letters, and the structured approach I have set out here can look a little daunting. Please don't be put off! Once you begin to write letters you may find that they naturally follow the flow I have outlined in this chapter. Indeed, this step-by-step process was developed by analysing actual letters people had written and seeing what was most helpful. The structure given here is only a suggestion, to provide you with some ways to stimulate your compassionate mind to help you. Indeed, many people have used the steps to help them in their compassion work without ever writing a single letter. For example, some people develop compassionate letters in their heads, but rather than write them down, dictate them to themselves or write compassionate poems or songs – even draw compassionate cartoons! Whatever works for you is absolutely fine; remember, the key is knowing what is helpful in the moment.

My personal reflections on Chapter 8

You might find it helpful to write down your key personal learning points from this chapter.

- How did you find the idea that you might need to compassionately tolerate distress?

- How could you make compassionate actions more of a habit?

- Do you think compassionate thought balancing or letter writing might help you on your journey to eating well and being less self-critical?

- Have you found your own ways of developing more compassionate thoughts, feelings and behaviours that you could use to help you learn to eat well?

SUMMARY

This chapter has explored why you might need to compassionately tolerate distress, at least for a short time, to help you learn
new ways to manage your feelings and thoughts. We explored
ways to act compassionately, even if you don't feel compassionate
towards yourself or others. Finally, we explored some techniques
to help you think more compassionately using compassionate
thought balancing and compassionate letter writing. Sometimes
it helps us to think more compassionately if we have an understanding of why we are responding to events or emotions in a
certain way. We call this a compassionate formulation. We will
explore this in more detail in the next chapter.

Thirteen steps to compassionate letter writing

Before beginning your letter, get into a compassionate mindset
by bringing your compassionate mind online. Allow yourself at
least half an hour to write your letter, and plan something soothing or distracting to do when you have finished.

1. Begin by getting in touch with the feelings or situations you
    are likely to find difficult. Do this by imagining yourself
    being in the situation you are going to face. Jot them down
    quickly – don't stay here for long!

2. Step outside the feelings using mindfulness or your soothing
    breathing rhythm.

3. Activate feelings of safety by developing your safe place.

4. Bring to mind your compassionate mind, in the form of your
    compassionate companion or 'you at your best'.

5. Begin your letter by recognising your courage, your resilience and the ways you have coped, both recently and in the past.

6. Develop empathy and understanding for your difficulties:

   - They are understandable – be specific about your history and memories of previous ways of coping, and the key threats that you were trying to avoid.

   - Understand the unintended consequences of your current ways of managing these difficulties.

   - Remind yourself that these events and ways of coping are not your fault, but they are your responsibility.

7. Consider what you need to help you cope with the difficulty.

   - What did I need in the past?

   - What do I need now?

8. Develop compassionate coping thoughts and behaviours to deal with the struggle differently.

9. Think about how your life would be different if you were able to be more self-compassionate.

10. Make a compassionate commitment to the changes you feel ready to make.

11. Pay compassionate attention to your letter:

    - Find your compassionate voice.

    - Reread your letter out loud to yourself. Ideally, use a mirror, or a photo.

12. Listen with your heart and wisdom to anything that could help your letter become even more compassionate.

13. Do something soothing or distracting when you finish your letter.

9 Understanding your current eating pattern

This chapter offers a very practical approach to making sense of the reasons that you overeat; by helping you learn ways to record when you do and do not eat well, and to look for patterns. We will explore how to use a diary to do this, the difficulties that many people have with using a diary (particularly if it gets hijacked by your critical or dieting mindset), and how to address blocks. In the next two chapters we will work with you to develop a here-and-now understanding of why you might find it difficult to eat well (Chapter 10), and why these difficulties may have developed based on your personal history (Chapter 11). The aim of these three chapters is to help you better understand your eating so that you can identify key patterns, thoughts and feelings to work on that will help you on your journey to eating well for the rest of your life.

Keeping an eating diary: a compassionate approach

An eating diary can help you learn to observe and become mindful of your eating patterns in a structured way. This can be a really helpful tool in changing your relationship with food but is often used by people in a dieting mindset to limit their eating or to beat themselves up when they break their eating rules. This chapter uses a compassionate approach to keeping an eating dairy, with the intention of helping you to understand what helps you eat well, and what gets in the way.

The main compassionate purposes of learning to monitor your eating habits, and the thoughts and emotions that affect them, are to:

- get an overview of your difficulties

- look for and make sense of patterns in triggers to overeating

- look for and make sense of things that protect you from overeating

- help slow down the 'inevitable' rush to overeat

- record your coping thoughts and strategies

- record and understand your progress in addressing overeating.

As for how to keep an eating diary, there are only two rules for monitoring your eating:

1. Do it in real time – as you eat or as soon as possible afterwards, not at the end of the day.

2. Be honest!

The amount of time it takes to get the hang of keeping a diary will vary from one person to another, but you'll probably want to spend several weeks or even a few months doing it so that you get a really good overview.

The diary in Worksheet 8 is a form that you can use to monitor your eating. Take a few moments to read through the headings. It might look a bit daunting at first, so after looking at it section by section we'll go through a real-life example using a day of Alison's diary.

Situation

The first column is designed to help you make sense of the circumstances that led up to overeating, or that protect us from either dieting or overeating.

Sometimes overeating can be triggered by being in particular places or is more common at different times of the year, month or day.

Some people can help us avoid overeating, while others may deliberately or accidentally encourage it. Some of our relationships can be difficult, and our emotions when we're with these people – or after we've been with them – can lead to overeating.

At this point there are two types of feelings we are interested in. The first is your *physical sensations*. These include whether you feel hungry or full, although if you have been dieting or overeating for some time, you may have lost touch with these bodily sensations, so it may not be easy to say at first. You can also record here whether you feel tired, restless, agitated, etc.

The other type of feeling we are interested in is your *emotions* – whether you feel anxious, sad, bored, angry, irritable or any of the many other possibilities. You may, of course, be feeling pleasant emotions, such as joy, pleasure or excitement. Commonly, we will be feeling a mixture or having rapid changes in our emotions.

As for what you're thinking, this too may not be easy to pinpoint at first. Sometimes we can be unaware of our thoughts, and it is a skill to be able to recognise them. You may find this easier as you get used to keeping your eating diary. If you do notice you are thinking in a particular way, or about particular things, this can give you a clue to what triggers your eating.

Worksheet 8: Eating diary

Date and time:

Situation	What did I eat or drink?	Overeating	Mindset when eating	Thoughts and feelings
Where were you? *Who were you with?* *How were you feeling?* *What were you thinking about before you ate?*	*(Amount and type)* **Physical activity** before or after eating *(Type and duration)*	Yes/No	*(e.g. dieting, comfort, food as fun, food as punishment)*	*These can be before, during or after eating, can be about doing the diary or anything else you think is important.*

We can break thinking down into three areas:

1. memories – positive or unpleasant – that you have before eating

2. thoughts about problems you are facing or going to face in the future

3. thoughts about eating, including the possible benefits of overeating or problems that overeating may create for you.

There may of course be other types of thoughts that you have that are not related to overeating, and it may be helpful to write these down too.

What you eat and/or drink, and what physical activity you take

In the second column, you can write what you are eating or drinking. Ideally you will also record roughly how much you have eaten – however, don't worry about recording or adding up calories at this point. You will only do this when you review your diary, and we'll explore how to do this a little later. This column will be very helpful for working out whether your overeating is actually related to your not giving your body enough food during the day. It may also help you notice whether any particular types of food are more likely to be associated with overeating. Remember that there are a number of 'non-foods' that are also associated with overeating. These include alcohol, medications and some illegal drugs. It is also important to list what and how much of these you take every day, to help you work out if they affect how much you eat.

It is also useful to keep a brief note of the types and amount of physical activity that you do – for example, noting down if you do an hour of housework, or go to the gym for thirty minutes each day, etc. The information in this column can help you to work out your energy and nutritional balance, and notice whether particular types of food trigger overeating.

Have you overeaten?

The third column asks you if you believe that you have overeaten. This is important, because sometimes we think that we have or haven't overeaten because of the types of food we eat or our feelings at the time, rather than as a result of an objective decision about what our body needed at a particular time, or how our eating compares to that of people who are more in touch with their bodies' needs and appetites.

What mindset are you in while you are eating?

The fourth column prompts you to consider what kind of mindset you are in when you are eating. This will help you to recognise what kind of eating you're doing and also to think about what problems this mindset is trying to help you manage. The main types we are interested in here are the ones that are most likely to influence your eating: the 'comfort food' and 'dieting' mindsets. However, you may also find that other types, such as being in an anxious, depressed or angry mindset, can also influence your overeating.

What are you thinking and feeling?

The final column explores your thoughts and feelings while you're eating and afterwards. In a more advanced version of this diary, you can also use this column to record thoughts, feelings or things you do that help you to manage your urges to overeat or to limit overeating. In your early diaries you may find that you have a lot of self-critical thoughts about overeating, or that it helps you to manage some difficult feelings.

Blocks to monitoring your eating

Monitoring may look like a pretty simple exercise – after all, it only has two rules: complete it in real time and be honest! In practice, many people find they come up against obstacles when they start trying to monitor their eating. These generally fall into one of two categories: practical or emotional.

Practical blocks include:

- difficulty in learning to use Worksheet 8

- difficulty in keeping the diary private

- problems completing it when other people are around

- finding the time to do it.

Emotional blocks include:

- resenting doing the task

- worrying that being more observant and mindful of your difficulties will make your eating or feelings worse

- seeing what you eat written down making you feel more self-critical or ashamed

- worrying about what others will think if they see you doing the diary

- triggering difficult memories of diary keeping (for example, if other people made you do this, and this led to criticism or feelings of shame).

Managing emotional blocks to monitoring

Practical blocks sound easier to address, but in fact are often more manageable once you have worked though emotional blocks. So, let's start with some of the most common of these.

The first emotional block for most people is finding a reason for keeping the diary that will prompt you to fill it in even if it is a struggle. We will explore motivation to change in Chapter 12, but for now you might try thinking of keeping a diary as a leap of faith – something that's worth a try to see if it can help you. Again, you may wish to explore the idea of keeping a diary from the perspective of your compassionate image. What would 'you at your best' or your compassionate companion say to help you take this leap of faith? How would they express their under-standing of and care for your real and honest concerns that the diary could be emotionally challenging for you? What would they say about the advantages for you personally? What kind of compassionate plan might they come up with to help you deal with your emotional blocks?

Many people worry that doing the diary will be upsetting, and this can happen, particularly as you begin to make connections between eating and your thoughts and feelings. However, this distress tends to be temporary, and it can remind you that what you're doing has a purpose: that if you can learn to tolerate a certain amount of distress now, you're likely to be better able to prevent yourself overeating in the future, and to learn new ways to manage your thoughts and feelings. Even so, keeping the diary short, not rereading it at the end of the day, or even keeping each eating episode written in a separate place (so you don't have to see your day's eating all in one go) can help you to avoid getting upset. You may also wish to plan soothing and distraction exercises to do after you have written your diary. By using whichever of these techniques suits you, you can put together a plan for making your diary emotionally manageable.

It's also important to make sure you review your diary from a compassionate mindset. Diaries can often be used by people as a way of beating themselves up for what they have eaten or why they eat – and this is absolutely *not* the idea here. Remember all that we discovered in the earlier chapters of this book about where our impulses and habits to do with eating come from – way back in our common ancestry and also in our early personal histories. The habits and practices you've been using are just the best ways you've found so far to deal with your own circumstances; what we're aiming to do now is to give you new and better ways to do this with information and understanding that you haven't had before.

Managing practical blocks to monitoring

The eating diary worksheet may look a bit cumbersome but many people get used to it fairly quickly and become happy to fill it in using this format. However, this is certainly not the only way to do it. Several people I have worked with prefer to keep the information in their own personal diaries; this can help the task to feel more private and special to you. By all means buy yourself a nice diary or notebook, ideally one that can be locked or is inconspicuous, to use as your monitoring record.

I have found that people can be really ingenious in managing this task. For example, texting the information to one's own mobile phone can be a good way both to get the information down quickly and to keep it private.

As for the time it takes, monitoring is designed to be done quite rapidly – I would suggest taking no more than a minute or so for each episode of eating. So, it shouldn't take any more than ten to fifteen minutes a day. It is important, however, not to leave this until the end of the day and do it all at once then. It really does help to have the information recorded at the time you're eating, or at least immediately afterwards. Most people can remember what they ate and when at the end of the day, but it's not so easy to remember accurately how you were feeling and what you were thinking at the time. You might want to use a personal code to note down your feelings and thoughts; this can be a good way to get the information down privately and quickly. Other ways of doing this are to record a few short lines as a phone message, in an email or on a scrap of paper. It doesn't matter how you get the information down, really, so long as you do it as soon as possible. If you end up with a collection of what seem like scrappy notes, you can always write up a 'neat' copy at the end of the day. A word of warning here, though: I suggest you try to do this fairly rapidly, because dwelling for too long on a whole day's eating, feelings and thoughts might leave you feeling a bit upset or uncomfortable.

It can be helpful to identify any of your own blocks to monitoring, and to try to find solutions to them, before you begin to keep your diary. Worksheet 9 overleaf is a form you can use to help you do this – or you can of course create your own. Figure 9.1 shows a completed example.

Worksheet 9: Managing blocks to monitoring eating

My personal blocks to monitoring my eating	Compassionate things I can say to myself or do to get past the block

Figure 9.1 Managing blocks to monitoring eating – an example

My personal blocks to monitoring eating	Compassionate things I can say to myself or do to get past the block
It brings attention to my overeating.	*It's understandable to feel a bit upset when I become aware of the difficulties – but in my heart I would like to move forward on this and so learning how to face my embarrassment or distress can be helpful in the long run. Maybe I can try it a few times and see how it goes.*
This is boring and I really don't like having to do these kinds of monitoring things.	*It's true, this can be boring, but maybe I could just have a couple of tries to get going and see how I do. Perhaps I could put a small note on the fridge to remind myself. To be honest, there are lots of things I do in my life that I find it boring, so this doesn't have to be a block. I am quite capable of doing boring things if I recognise they can be helpful in the long run.*
I guess I feel bad because I'm being quite critical really – I don't like myself because of my overeating.	*I should remember that this is not my fault. I have a see-food-and-eat-it brain – and the food industry has encouraged me to want certain foods. I also learned to use eating to support myself emotionally because it helped at the time. It's more important to be kind and understanding and recognise that there is a problem here and that if I go gently and kindly with myself, I can begin to find new ways forward.*

Using your diary to make sense of your eating

Once you've got used to keeping your eating diary, you can start using Worksheet 10 to draw together the information you've collected and start to identify the things that protect you from, as well as those that put you at risk of, overeating. Again, it is important when you review your diary that you do so from the perspective of your compassionate mind, exploring the patterns you find in a genuine spirit of concerned curiosity, wanting to understand and then find ways to alleviate the uncomfortable and perhaps painful emotions that your overeating both helps you with and causes for you. It's also a good idea to set aside time to soothe any distress the reviewing process causes.

Worksheet 10: Eating diary review

Eating pattern

How long do I leave between each eating episode?

How many times per day do I eat more often than every 3–4 hours?

How many times per day do I eat less than every 3–4 hours?

Energy needs

What is my daily energy need (calories)?

How much energy do I take in each day (calories)?

Am I eating more or less than I need each day?

What I eat and drink

Are there specific types of food that trigger overeating – if so, what are they?

Are there any foods that help me to not overeat?

Are there any things I take into my body that affect my appetite or eating (e.g. medication, drugs, alcohol)?

Times, people, places

Are there any times, people or places that make overeating more likely?

Are there any times, people or places that protect me from overeating?

My feelings and overeating

Are there any feelings that make overeating more likely/worse?

Are these physical sensations, such as hunger?

Are there emotions, such as sadness, boredom, anger, anxiety?

My thoughts and overeating

Am I in dieting mindset before, during or after overeating?

Am I in comfort food mindset before, during or after overeating?

Do I give myself permission to overeat as a 'treat'?

Do I use overeating to punish myself?

Do I hope that overeating will help me manage difficult feelings, memories or events?

Do I follow certain rules or habits that I have been taught about eating?

Do I criticise myself about what I have eaten or the way that I eat?

Am I worried about what other people think about my overeating?

If you answer 'yes' to any of these questions, try to be as specific as you can about exactly what you are thinking and, if you can, how and when you learned to think this way.

When I review diaries with my clients, we put aside at least an hour at the end of the week and review a whole week's worth. This gives us a much better idea of patterns; indeed, sometimes we will review four weeks' worth of diaries together to get a longer-term perspective. It can take a week or two to get the hang of keeping the diary, so you might want to wait until you feel you have a week's worth of complete daily records before you can start your review.

As we have seen in previous chapters, there is a whole range of factors that can affect your eating habits. They include the following.

Eating pattern

As we found in Chapter 2, eating patterns can significantly affect our risk of overeating. When looking at your diary, it is important to look for the spaces between eating episodes. Your body can last for about three or four hours before it starts getting hungry. Eating more frequently than this can put us out of touch with our hunger, while leaving longer gaps puts us at risk of overeating at the next meal.

Energy balance

As we also saw in Chapter 2, our bodies need a certain amount of energy just to keep our physical systems going; and we need a variable amount on top of this to fuel whatever we do during the day. If we overeat, we can lose touch with our bodily needs; if, on the other hand, we are trying to eat less than our body needs we are likely to overeat – as well as to experience a range of psychological and physical side effects. So, what we're aiming for is an 'energy balance': eating just the right amount to support our physical systems and our activities.

Many people who overeat will be quite good at estimating their energy intake, although they may be less aware of the amount they use or need. Unless you have access to a dietitian who can work this out for you, this is a skill that you will need to develop. We'll explore how to do this in more detail in Chapter 13, but it's worth taking a look at the basic principles here.

The easiest (but by no means easy) way to estimate your energy intake is to become familiar with the calorie content of what you eat and drink. There are many commercial calorie-counting books, websites and apps that can help you to do this. You might find adding up your calorie intake an uncomfortable exercise at first; try to view it as a necessary step in helping you to gain control over your eating, and support yourself compassionately while you do it.

Our energy needs depend on our body weight, height, energy use and gender. We will explore this in more detail in Chapter 13. It is normal to have a variation of about 200–300 calories a day – your body is more than capable of adjusting to this – but your overall aim is a balance in your energy over the week. You can skip ahead to Chapter 13 if you want to work out your energy needs now, but as this can be upsetting for some people you may wish to keep reading each chapter in turn until you get there naturally.

Keeping an eye on your calorie intake to try to establish an appropriate energy balance can really help you to tackle overeating. It is likely that if you are using this book to help you eat well you may find it difficult to balance your energy at this stage. Don't worry; we will work on how to do this in more detail in Chapter 15.

What you eat and drink

Many people find that specific types of food act as a trigger to overeating. These may be foods that we associate with comfort, that are 'forbidden' in some way, or that we simply really like! Learning to eat and enjoy these in moderation can be really important in managing overeating.

Times, people, places

Often, overeating happens in a regular or predictable way – for example, many of us overeat at weekends, or when we are with others who overeat. Understanding these patterns can help us plan to manage these situations.

Your feelings and overeating

As we explored earlier, it can be helpful to divide feelings into *physical sensations* (including hunger) and *emotions* (such as anger, boredom or anxiety), although of course these are often mingled together. It can sometimes be difficult to identify both kinds of feeling, particularly if eating helps you to manage them. Sometimes you may have to delay responding to the urge to overeat for a little while to be able to identify your feelings more clearly. We explored how to do this in Chapter 8. Once you can identify these feelings, you are on your way to learning to understand and manage them in a more compassionate way.

Your thoughts and overeating

There are many ways in which our thoughts can lead to overeating. They can:

* give us positive permission to overeat, telling us for example that we 'deserve food' because we have been good or had a hard time

* allow us to punish ourselves with food

- encourage us to hope that eating will help us to manage unpleasant feelings or experiences

- encourage, support or bully us into dieting, and thus increase our risk of overeating later

- provide rules that lead to accidental or habitual overeating (such as 'I must always clear my plate').

Our thoughts are also very likely to be intertwined with our feelings. Sometimes they have less to with eating itself than with how we think about ourselves, or how we think other people will think about us after we have overeaten, or if they find out that we overeat. These patterns can lead us into vicious cycles of secret eating or dieting.

Our thoughts can also help us to manage our urges to overeat or to cope when we have overeaten. Validating, supporting and encouraging the thoughts that help us is a major step in controlling overeating. Your diary can help you to identify and build upon these thoughts, and to develop new ones.

One cautionary note: I encourage my clients not to review their diary if they have had a particularly difficult day, nor to do it just before they go to bed, when they will probably be tired and tempted to brood critically on what they have recorded rather than analyse it compassionately. It is better to do the review when feeling relatively calm, alert and able to learn from our diaries.

Making sense of Alison's diary

In the final section of this chapter, we will review a sample day from Alison's diary (Figure 9.2) to give you an idea of how reviewing a diary works in practice, and how what you learn can help you to beat overeating for good.

Figure 9.2 Alison's eating diary

Date and time: Monday 23 March

Situation	What did I eat or drink?	Overeating	Mindset when eating	Thoughts and feelings
Where were you? Who were you with? How were you feeling? What were you thinking about before you ate?	(Amount and type) Physical activity before or after eating (Type and duration)	Yes/No	(e.g. dieting, comfort, food as fun, food as punishment)	These can be before, during or after eating, can be about doing the diary or anything else you think is important.
8 a.m. At home, alone. A bit tired and hungry. Not really thinking about anything.	Cereal, 2 slices of toast and butter. Cup of tea, skimmed milk no sugar.	No	No mindset was active.	Felt OK about eating. Worried about going to work today.
10 a.m. At work with colleagues. Worried about difficult meeting later today.	Cup of tea with skimmed milk and 5 ginger biscuits.	Yes	Comfort food mindset.	Felt a bit worried that colleagues would think I was greedy, but felt I needed the food to calm me down.

Time, place, situation	Food and drink	Binge?	Mindset	Feelings
11.30 p.m. At work. Alone. Felt a bit queasy, not hungry. More anxious about the meeting at noon.	Tea with skimmed milk and 10 biscuits. Had planned to have lunch but couldn't face it. Left the office and went for 10-minute walk.	Yes	Comfort food mindset when eating. Planned to not eat biscuits for the rest of the week. Dieting mindset.	Felt greedy and ashamed about eating.
1.45 p.m. At a restaurant alone. Very upset by the meeting, felt angry with my boss and useless. Mainly thinking about the meeting and what other people thought about me.	Burger meal. Large milkshake.	No	Comfort food mindset. Planning not to eat for the rest of the day.	Felt OK about eating but very down and critical of myself. Worried about going back to work.
6 p.m. No planned evening meal.	Cup of coffee with skimmed milk.	No	Dieting mindset.	Very upset about meeting and overeating earlier.
10.30 p.m. Home with partner. Still upset about work. Felt I deserved a treat as the day was so hard.	4 glasses of red wine. Takeaway meal plus partner's leftovers (4 slices of pizza). Individual tub of ice cream.	Yes	Dieting mindset just before meal, but partner came in late with a takeaway – 'food as fun' and comfort food mindsets.	Didn't want to eat, felt out of control when I started to eat and could not stop. Angry with myself for overeating. Planning to eat a lot less tomorrow.

Usually, the more information we have the easier it is to make sense of a diary, so it's a good idea to review a whole week's records together. There may also be monthly or seasonal patterns to our relationship with overeating that we only see when we look at a much longer period. However, even looking at one day can be very revealing – and that's what we're going to do here.

Alison used the eating diary review worksheet as a guide to help her make sense of the information from her eating diary. When we review her diary, we see that four of her eating episodes occurred relatively close together (at 8 a.m., 10 a.m., 12.30 p.m. and 1.45 p.m.) but that there was then a very long gap until her final meal of the day at 10.30 p.m. On reflection, she noticed that she wasn't particularly hungry at 10 a.m. or 12.30 p.m., but in the evening had been fending off feeling hungry from about 6 p.m. By looking over a lot of similar days' records, Alison became aware of a couple of issues that she decided to work on. The first was learning to eat when her body was more likely to be hungry, and to avoid eating when she didn't need to, even if that meant not eating at times when other people were. The second was a long-standing pattern – which in fact amounted to a 'rule' – that she should not eat in the evening. This left her feeling deprived, hungry and likely to overeat if she did break her rule.

Alison also noticed that other people being around and being on her own both increased her risk of overeating in different ways. She found it hard not to overeat when she was with work colleagues, or if her partner offered her food to cheer her up. However, when she was alone, she also tended to comfort eat. Alison was able to identify both anxiety and anger as feelings that she managed by using food.

Before starting to keep a diary, Alison believed that she overate all the time. She was surprised to find that some of her meals (e.g. breakfast) were actually normal portions. Later on, when she worked out her energy intake for this day, she found that she had eaten at least 1,500 calories more than her body needed. This wasn't really news to Alison, although she did find it upsetting to see it written down. What was more interesting was that at lunchtime she couldn't face eating the sandwich, bag of crisps and apple she'd taken to work because it felt like overeating – but actually these added up to fewer calories than the biscuits that she ate instead.

As she thought more about what she'd eaten on this day, Alison remembered that she had always been offered biscuits to help her manage being upset when she was growing up. This helped her to think about the urge to eat biscuits being a good warning sign that she might need to deal with her feelings, as well as to focus on eating foods that would be more filling, like her sand-wich and crisps (even if they felt too fattening), to help her avoid overeating later.

The final thing she realised was that alcohol tended to make her feel hungrier and less able to control her urges to overeat. This helped her to think about changing her drinking habits, and in particular trying to reduce the amount of alcohol she drank if she was upset, anxious or angry.

Alison was particularly skilled in recognising the mindsets she was in when she was eating. She fluctuated between her 'comfort food' and her 'dieting' mindsets. These often clouded her whole day but also helped her to deal with threatening events – for example, the distressing meeting she had at work on this day. Thinking about food in one way or another helped her to avoid thinking about the meeting for large parts of the day. She was also able to notice that she often struggled with feeling greedy after eating, became worried about what other people thought about her if they saw her eating, and could get very angry with herself when she overate. She noticed that her anger was helpful in fuelling her urges to diet and to avoid being seen as greedy, and in preventing her from overeating later, but often led to her feeling even worse and needing to comfort eat to manage this.

It took Alison several weeks of diary keeping to identify these patterns clearly, and some time after that to decide which areas to work on first in trying gradually to reduce her overeating. In the next chapter, we will explore how you can use the information from your diary to develop a compassionate understanding of your own difficulties and to set realistic goals for addressing your overeating.

My personal reflections on Chapter 9

You might find it helpful to write down your key personal learning points from this chapter.

- What were your first thoughts about keeping a diary of your eating and activity?

- What ways have you found to help you with any blocks to diary keeping?

- What did you learn from reviewing your first week of diaries?

SUMMARY

This chapter has explored a practical way of recording and exploring the patterns and triggers than may influence your current eating habits. In Chapter 10, we will put this information together to help you develop a personal understanding of your eating and how your eating habits help you to regulate your threat system or access your drive and soothing systems. We will also explore the intended and unintended consequences of not eating well.

10 How does your eating work now?

In the previous chapter we explored how keeping an eating diary can help you to become more observant of your overeating, and how you can begin to make sense of the information you gather in this way by reviewing your diary.

It's worth pausing here to repeat that if you're struggling to deal with overeating, you are certainly not alone: overeating is a problem for over half of the Western world. Nor does it mean that there is anything wrong with *you*. Overeating is likely to be the outcome of the complex interactions between your genetic make-up, biological mechanisms that helped us all successfully survive famine, and events in your own life that have either taught you to overeat or that overeating could help you in some way.

In the first three chapters we explored these mechanisms in some detail and introduced the 'three systems' approach to understanding how we regulate our emotions. In this chapter and the next we will explore ways to help you make sense of why you overeat and the impact this may have on you. In turn, this can give you clues about the thoughts, feelings, emotions or habits you may need to work on to help you eat well.

Overeating and the 'three systems' of emotional regulation

The 'three systems' model of emotional regulation can be a very helpful way of thinking about how our overeating can affect or be used (deliberately or accidentally) to manage our emotional life.

As you may remember, we are interested in three main systems:

1. the *threat system*, which is mainly about helping to stop us doing, or get us away from, things that we believe are unpleasant or dangerous to us; the main emotions in this system include fear/anxiety, anger and disgust

2. the *drive system*, which is concerned with helping us reach specific goals; the main emotions in this system are excitement, celebration and pride

3. the *soothing system*, which focuses on making us feel calm, soothed and cared for.

We need all three systems to help us manage the challenges of life; and all of them can be affected by, and can in turn affect, the eating habits we learn and get used to. As we have seen, feeling soothed by food ('the comfort food mind') can replace other ways of feeling cared for and contented. The 'dieting mind' is often connected with the drive/achievement system, so that dieting can feel like an achievement in itself and a way to get closer to other goals we have in life. Both mindsets can be turned on when we feel under threat in some way, either externally (things that are happening to us) or internally (from our memories, thoughts and feelings). Often a threat has elements of both types. Once our threat/protection system is active, we tend to see things that we would normally feel OK about as threats too. Do remember that this rapid escalation of the threat system is perfectly normal: after all, it evolved to protect us, and it wouldn't have been much good at that if it had been easy to ignore! But because it is so active and so powerful, it can quickly become difficult for us to see the wood for the trees, as we seem to be surrounded by threats and under pressure to respond to or retreat from them. So, it can be helpful to work out in advance what things trigger the system, and then what additional issues arise once it has got into its stride.

In a compassionate mind approach to eating well, we are particularly interested in helping you work out whether the balance between these three systems has become skewed. We also want to see if 'comfort food' or 'dieting', or other overeating mindsets (e.g. 'eating for fun' or 'eating to belong'), have got entangled with these systems. Finally, we want to see if the ways you have been using to try to manage these systems have had unintentional side effects that are making it even more difficult for you.

In the next section of this chapter, we will explore how overeating may help you to manage your three emotional regulation systems. This will provide you with a deeper understanding of how eating helps you in the here and now.

This analysis revolves around nine questions that help us to make sense of the reasons why we overeat and the unintended consequences:

1. Am I at greater risk of overeating when my threat system comes online?

2. What types of threat emotions are most likely to trigger my overeating?

3. Are there any other threats that I pay attention to once my threat system is active?

4. How does eating help me to cope when my threat system is switched on?

5. Does eating help me to feel soothed?

6. Does eating help me turn off or tone down my threat system?

7. Does eating activate my drive system?

8. What do I hope that eating will make me feel (the intended consequence of eating)?

9. What are the unintended consequences of overeating?

We will work through Alison's responses to these nine questions to show you how they can help guide your exploration.

Alison's analysis of her eating and the three systems

Using her eating diary (part of which we looked at in Chapter 9), Alison began to develop her analysis of how her overeating related to her three emotional systems, taking the nine key questions in turn – sometimes one at a time and sometimes in groups, starting with the first three questions.

Key questions:

1. Am I at greater risk of overeating when my threat system comes online?

2. What types of threat emotions are most likely to trigger my overeating?

3. Are there any other threats that I pay attention to once my threat system is active?

Looking back at the diary entry she completed for Monday 23 March, Alison noticed that the day's biggest trigger to overeating was the meeting just before lunchtime with her boss. This was a routine meeting to review her work performance. Alison wanted to use it to make her boss aware that she had taken on a lot of work recently that was beyond both her pay grade and her training. She had spent a lot of time planning how to let her boss know that she was upset about this additional burden and wanted them to reduce the demands made on her. However, Alison had found it difficult to be assertive with her employers in the past and already expected that they would do nothing to rectify the situation. Alison recognised that her problems with assertiveness cropped up in many relationships and believed that they dated back to her childhood. She noticed that both anticipated and actual experiences of wanting to be assertive with others tended to activate her threat system.

Alison also noticed that when her threat system was in play, she was likely to remember times in her life when her needs had not been met by others. She was also likely to be angry with herself for finding it difficult to be assertive.

Key questions:

4. How does eating help me to cope when my threat system is switched on?

5. Does eating help me to feel soothed?

6. Does eating help me turn off or tone down my threat system?

Alison noticed that eating helped her to deal with feelings about the meeting in several ways. First, the food helped to soothe her anxiety. She also noticed that the types of food she ate reminded her of people who had cared for her. For example, the smell of the ginger biscuits she ate at 10 a.m. reminded her of her grand-mother, who used to bake with her when she was growing up.

Alison also found that focusing on the taste and pleasure of eating her burger helped to take her mind off the meeting after it happened. It also temporarily distracted her from self-critical thoughts about her performance in the meeting.

Key question:

7.   Does eating activate my drive system?

Some people who overeat are proud of their ability to eat more than others. There are even world records for the most hotdogs you can eat! However, for most people this is not the way their drive system is activated when they overeat. More usually, it is either anticipation of the pleasure of eating or planning to diet that will activate it.

Alison had both of these experiences. She had not planned to have a burger and milkshake for lunch that day – indeed, she had actually brought in a sandwich. But once the meeting was over, she told herself that she deserved something nice to eat because she had survived what she thought would be a very difficult meeting (in fact, her boss had praised some of her work and was not as critical as she had predicted). She spent the hour between finishing the meeting and her lunch break anticipating the flavours of her favourite food and the pleasure it would bring her.

Once she had finished eating her burger, she then spent a lot of time thinking about how she needed to diet to manage the extra food she had eaten that day. She remembered the times she had dieted and lost a little weight in the past, and the sense of achievement that eating less would bring her.

As we can see, the drive system can be turned on by the things we actually do, but a lot of the time the focus is on how we will feel when we have achieved our goals: to this extent it can often be driven as much by hope and wanting as by actually getting what we want.

Key question:

8.   What do I hope that eating will make me feel (the intended consequence of eating)?

Alison hoped that eating would both calm her anxiety and reward her for facing a difficult situation. She gave herself permission to overeat by telling herself that she would diet later. Planning her diet also helped reduce her anxiety and manage her self-criticism by giving her something else to focus on. She also hoped that dieting would make her happier in the longer term, particularly as it helped to boost her self-confidence.

Key question:

9.   What are the unintended consequences of overeating?

This question took Alison a little more time to explore. She noticed that although eating did help her feel a little less anxious, after overeating she often felt greedy and out of control (i.e. self-critical) and worried that other people would also think that about her. Alison was worried about the effect of overeating on her health, but this concern tended to be less important than managing her fear of being criticised when her threat system was more active.

On further reflection, Alison noticed that although eating helped her to reduce her anxiety before the meeting, it meant that she had given less thought to how she was going to be assertive with her boss, or to addressing this very important issue in her life in the longer term. And, afterwards, her focus on rewarding herself with food for surviving the encounter meant that she didn't really compassionately listen to her sadness for the impact that not being assertive had had on her life, or make sense of her anger and grief for having her needs ignored for so long.

Your own analysis of eating and the three systems

Having read Alison's analysis, you may now wish to develop your own. You can use the information you have gathered from your diary as well as any other observations you (or other people) have made about your eating, to help you answer the nine questions.

The questions are set out in Worksheet 11, along with some brief comments that may help you answer them. Before you start, once again spend a few moments bringing your soothing system and then your compassionate mind online so that you are looking at these questions from a compassionate frame of mind, with a genuine curiosity based on a desire to understand in order to be helpful – not critical. Now spend some time writing out your own thoughts on each of the questions.

Worksheet 11: How my eating works now

1. Am I at greater risk of overeating when my threat system comes online?

If so, what ideas do you have about why this might happen?

2. What types of threat emotions are most likely to trigger my overeating?

Try to think about what reasons there may be for this, perhaps by thinking about your personal history or current circumstances.

3. Are there any other threats that I pay attention to once my threat system is active?

Often when our threat system comes online, we can end up in 'threat spirals', feeling more and more threatened. This type of threat escalation is very normal. It can be useful to identify any new types of threats that emerge and how your eating may help you deal with them as well as with the original threat that was triggered.

4. How does eating help me to cope when my threat system is switched on?

For example, do you feel more in control of things when you are eating or planning a diet?

5. Does eating help me to feel soothed?

If you feel it does, think about in what way it does this; for example, does it help you to feel calm, bring in other soothing memories, etc.?

6. Does eating help me turn off or tone down my threat system?

For example, does it help you feel less anxious or numb? If so, how do you think eating does this?

7. Does eating activate my drive system?

For example, is it linked to having fun, or does compensating for overeating by dieting give you a feeling of pride or achievement?

8. What do I hope that eating will make me feel (the intended consequence of eating)?

For example, will it help you manage difficult situations, relationships or feelings? Does it tone down self-criticism or negative feelings about your body?

9. What are the unintended consequences of overeating?

For example, does it lead to feelings of guilt or shame later; does it impact on your relationships, daily activities or health?

Sometimes it is helpful to do this exercise several times, to help us explore the different threats that eating helps us with. For example, Alison could have worked through one worksheet to help her explore her feelings of being criticised by people she worked with, and another to explore concerns she had about upsetting other people in her life. If there were any differences between the two analyses, this might have suggested approaches she could take to managing the key threats she experienced and the safety strategies she used.

A compassionate formulation

A compassionate formulation is made up of four elements:

1. *key threats,* and the past and present influences that activate them

2. *safety strategies,* which can be used to provide us with a sense of external or internal safety

3. *intended consequences* of our safety strategies

4. *unintended consequences* of our safety strategies.

You can see this illustrated in Figure 10.1. Now this is a great model, but it is really hard to think about all of your relationships with food at once. To make it easier we focus on a particular situation – for example, overeating late in the evening. Then we break this down into different types of late-night eating (your diary can help you here), perhaps looking at overeating when you are bored. You can then repeat the exercise for all of the other times when you overeat in the evening (e.g. when you are alone, with others, when you are tired, when you have eaten a lot/very little during the day). This can help you to understand how each type of overeating works and to develop a plan to address them.

You may discover you need different solutions. We will explore this model in more detail in the next section.

Figure 10.1 A compassionate formulation

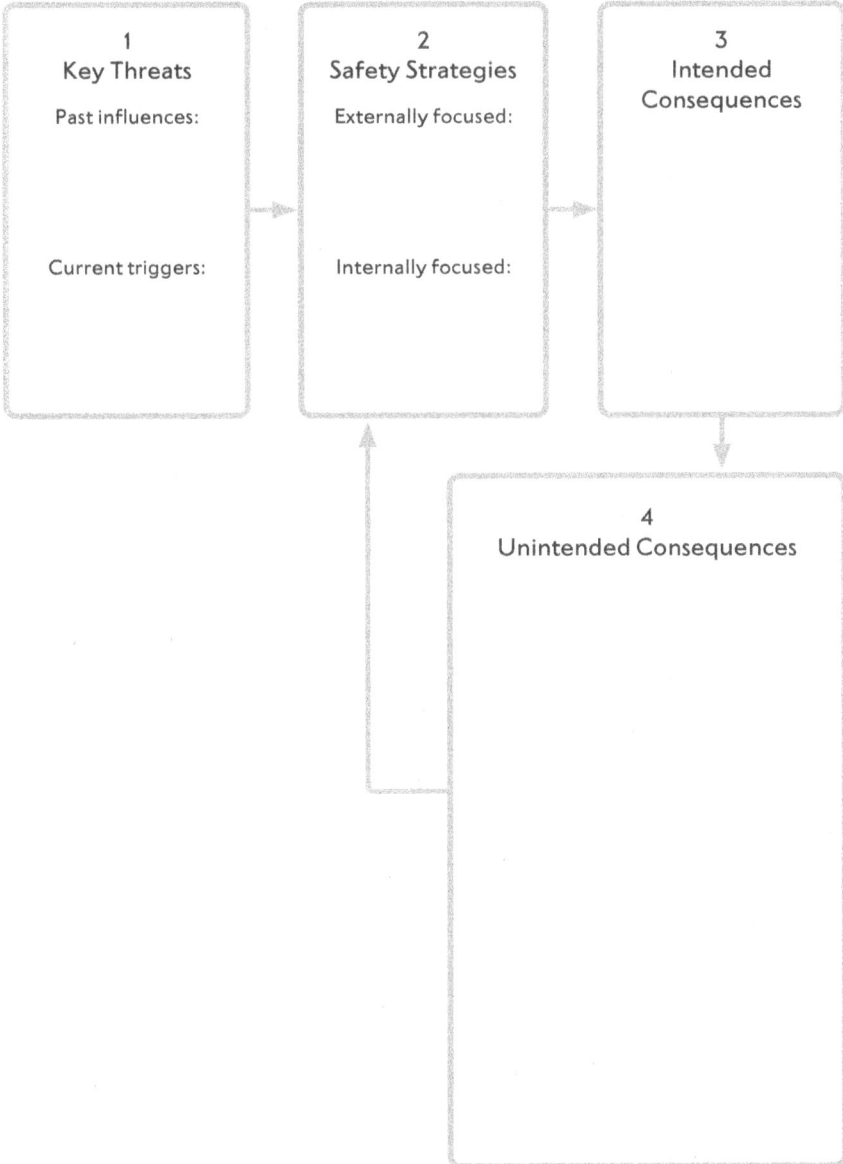

| 1
Key Threats

Past influences:

Current triggers: | 2
Safety Strategies

Externally focused:

Internally focused: | 3
Intended
Consequences |

| 4
Unintended Consequences |

Eating as a safety strategy

We create safety strategies to deal with things in our internal world – things that go on in our own heads, such as avoiding difficult emotions or trying to stimulate pleasurable emotions – and of course things that go on in the outside world, such as trying to avoid rejection, or getting people to like us and be kind to us. We call these *intended consequences*. The trouble is that the safety strategies we come up with as solutions can also become part of the problem. For example, imagine the difficulties some-body who's always submissive is going to run into, or those that will challenge somebody who never wants to confront an uncomfortable emotion. So, safety strategies can have *unintended consequences* too.

Now, as we have already seen, we may overeat or diet, and find our weight going up and down like a yo-yo, because, for example:

- we don't know enough about the way our eating patterns affect our weight

- the things that we consume other than food affect our appetite and our ability to regulate it

- of habits we learned while we were growing up.

Overeating can also be a *safety strategy*, which can serve a very useful purpose in helping us to regulate our emotions, and par-ticularly to manage the things that bother us most – our 'key threats', if you like. When overeating has become a way of deal-ing with our emotions it's important to recognise this, because if we're going to have a good chance of succeeding in changing our eating habits, we're going to need to work on the issues that drive it. For example, if we have an underlying sense of shame or of being out of control, simply trying to change our eating behaviour without changing those feelings may be tricky. Indeed, when we begin to challenge and work on our safety strategies, some of the key threats they were designed to deal with can resurface – so we're going to have to deal with them!

As the term implies, *safety strategies* are designed to keep us safe in some way. They can be deliberate and thought out, but they can also be things that we find ourselves doing without really knowing why. They fall into two categories: *external* (aimed at managing how other people will see us or treat us) and *internal* (about managing our own emotions and how we think or feel about ourselves).

Figure 10.1 shows you how safety strategies are developed in response to 'key threats', both past and present; how they have both intended and unintended consequences; and how these consequences keep the safety strategies in use. We can call the overall pattern a 'compassionate formulation for overeating'. To give you a better idea of how this works in practice, we're now going to look at Alison's formulation, which is summarised in Figure 10.2.

Figure 10.2 Alison's compassionate formulation for eating

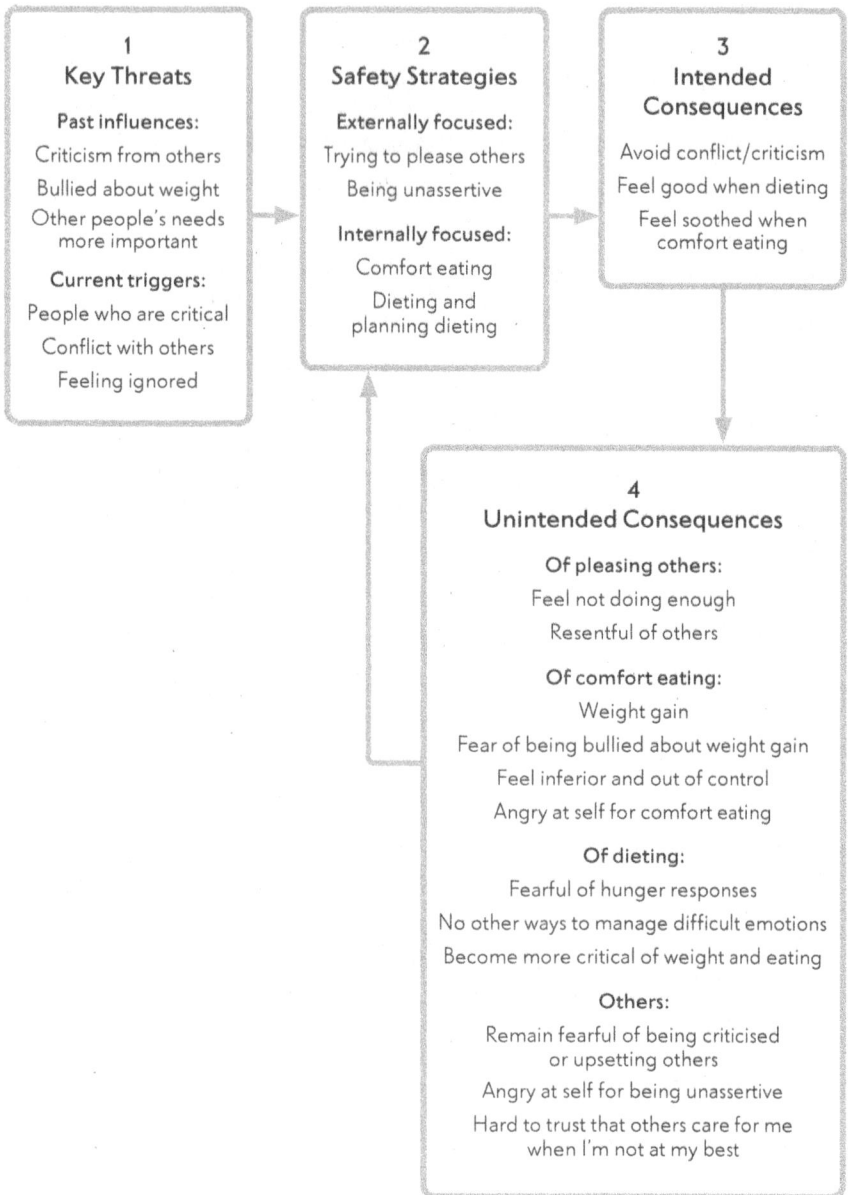

1
Key Threats

Past influences:
Criticism from others
Bullied about weight
Other people's needs
more important

Current triggers:
People who are critical
Conflict with others
Feeling ignored

2
Safety Strategies

Externally focused:
Trying to please others
Being unassertive

Internally focused:
Comfort eating
Dieting and
planning dieting

3
Intended
Consequences

Avoid conflict/criticism
Feel good when dieting
Feel soothed when
comfort eating

4
Unintended Consequences

Of pleasing others:
Feel not doing enough
Resentful of others

Of comfort eating:
Weight gain
Fear of being bullied about weight gain
Feel inferior and out of control
Angry at self for comfort eating

Of dieting:
Fearful of hunger responses
No other ways to manage difficult emotions
Become more critical of weight and eating

Others:
Remain fearful of being criticised
or upsetting others
Angry at self for being unassertive
Hard to trust that others care for me
when I'm not at my best

Exploring Alison's compassionate formulation for eating

Key threats: past influences

Alison recalls that when she was growing up her parents were very loving but set quite high standards for her. They were difficult to please and appeared disappointed if she failed at things. They were busy people. She remembers dreading any criticism intruding on the precious moments of loving attention or pride she had from them. She doesn't recall much open discussion of her feelings in any depth, learning that in life you 'just get on with things'. She also remembers that she had to work quite hard to succeed at things, as she was not a naturally gifted student.

So, Alison developed a belief that people liked and cared about you if you weren't a nuisance to them and just got on with and achieved things. She was very anxious about what other people thought about her when she couldn't do this. She felt that others saw her as a disappointment and would want to distance themselves from her rather than help if she failed or made mistakes.

Sadly, the belief that love, approval or support will be offered to us only if we 'deserve' them is a lot more common than most of us imagine. Many of us worry that if we struggle or fall over few genuine helping hands will come to our aid.

We can think about the beliefs Alison developed in terms of the three systems of emotional regulation that we discussed in Chapter 3 (you might want to look back at Figure 3.1 on page 67). Alison's sense of security has come to be based upon her ability to maintain her drive system. Only then does she begin to feel safe and less fearful of others. She doesn't find it easy to get access to her soothing system (through being kind to herself or expecting others to be kind to her).

Key threats: current triggers

By exploring her personal history, Alison came to recognise that as an adult she found it very difficult to deal with being criticised, or with situations where she might be. She found conflict very difficult and struggled to be assertive about her needs. She also noticed that feeling other people had overlooked or ignored her left her feeling angry towards them.

Alison began to recognise that one of the reasons why she didn't like any kind of conflict and could easily feel overwhelmed by it was that she had different feelings going on at the same time. For example, she was clearly anxious about the rejection of being put down, but there was also an element of anger in the background because she wanted to defend herself – and yet she was also anxious about this anger in case other people would see her as silly. So, she also tended to criticise herself for feeling angry. You won't be surprised to hear that anger was a feeling Alison struggled with and tried to avoid. So, you can probably guess what she did if she got angry – she ate.

Safety strategies

Alison saw that she had tried to avoid conflict and criticism mainly by trying to predict the needs of others, especially those in authority or who had some power over her, and to please them. Typically, she found that if the emotional temperature in a potential conflict was rising, she would immediately get anxious and back off, falling into a submissive attitude. That safety strategy was so well rehearsed that it was automatic for her, and even though she found herself battling with it at times she was also frightened to overrule it. She also recognised how both comfort eating and dieting had helped her to manage the threat of criticism.

So, Alison noticed that she had three main safety strategies, which she called 'pleasing others', 'comfort eating' and 'dieting'. Pleasing others is an example of an external safety strategy. Comfort eating was an internal safety strategy, designed to help Alison cope with or turn off painful feelings. Dieting was both an external safety strategy (helping her to manage her fear of criticism from others) and an internal safety strategy (helping to improve her feelings about herself and to give her a sense of achievement).

Intended consequences

The main consequences Alison intended from dieting were feeling better about herself and avoiding distressing thoughts about feeling inferior, out of control, criticised or in conflict with others. Comfort eating had the intended consequences of helping her to deal with distressing emotions (particularly anger) when these thoughts did arise, by soothing her. Being unassertive helped her to avoid conflict with and criticism from others.

Unintended consequences

Let's look at the unintended consequences of Alison's safety strategies in more detail. It is common for these consequences, which we don't plan or foresee, to maintain or even worsen our difficulties.

Pleasing others

Alison found that pleasing others covered a number of things she did to avoid being criticised. These included overworking, trying to predict and meet the needs of others, always putting her needs second, being unassertive and avoiding conflict. The unintended

consequences were that she felt harried, put upon, never achieving quite enough, somehow a failure and inadequate, yet also
resentful of the demands that others put on her and the effects
that meeting their needs had on her physical, emotional and
social life.

Comfort eating

Alison noticed that comfort eating really helped her to soothe her
distress (an intended consequence). Looking back, this pattern
had begun relatively early in her life and may have contributed
to her being slightly overweight between the ages of ten and
sixteen (an unintended consequence). She worried that gaining
weight through comfort eating would lead to her being bullied
again, and these worries often brought back the memories, and
associated distress, of the times when she had been bullied about
her weight in the past. As her weight increased her mood would
dip. The self-critical voice within her would start up again and
she would be angry with herself for being unable to control her
urges to eat.

Dieting

Alison remembered that dieting was initially a way of losing
some weight to avoid being bullied, and of giving herself a feeling of being in control and, to some degree, a sense of pride and
pleasure in her appearance. Her plans to diet would be triggered
by becoming more aware than usual of her weight and shape
(noticing, for example, that her jeans and dresses were getting
tight), and more critical of her appearance. However, she also
found it difficult to cope with feeling hungry and would get
angry with herself when she was tempted to break her diet.

When Alison was dieting she could not turn to comfort eating to cope with difficult emotions in her life. This meant that feelings of anger and irritation with herself (either because of her weight or at being hungry) were with her even more. Alison found that planning a diet could give her hope about managing her weight and distracted her temporarily. But then thoughts about dieting tended to intrude at other times in her life, for example, when she was trying to concentrate on tasks at work. Often she would find herself seeking reassurance from her partner that her diet was working – which he found quite irritating!

All safety strategies

Alison recognised that, together, her safety strategies had the unintended consequence of not allowing her to develop other ways to manage her fear of being criticised, her inability to assert herself and her anger and irritation towards others. She also noticed that she was often angry or disappointed with herself for needing to comfort eat, diet, or avoid conflict and criticism, and that this tended to lower her mood, even when she had supportive friends or family around her. This all left Alison feeling even more distressed and needing her safety strategies even more to help her to cope with her emotions.

Working out this 'formulation' of threats, safety strategies and intended and unintended consequences helped Alison to understand where her tendency to overeat had come from, but, more importantly, it helped her to make sense of why it had been so difficult to give it up over the years, despite really wanting to.

Having got to this point, Alison could begin to offer herself compassion for the pain she had experienced in the past and to recognise that overeating had been the best way she could help herself cope with that pain and to function in the world. Having compassionately acknowledged this, she could go on to explore new ways to address her key fears without using her old safety strategies and so work towards breaking out of the vicious circle of overeating.

Why draw up a compassionate formulation for eating?

It's important to think through why we want to set out a formulation like this, and how it relates to the compassionate mind approach we've discussed in earlier chapters of this book. We begin with a genuine desire to develop wisdom and insight into our difficulties. The process of building our formulation allows us to stand back and see how different pieces of our lives fit together. Alison could see how the difficulties she got into arose from the combination of her experiences in life and that she was likely to become even more stuck in her current vicious circle if she went on criticising and blaming herself for her difficulties and how she coped with them.

To sum up, setting out a compassionate formulation for our overeating helps us to:

- be open and honest without blaming ourselves

- recognise that our overeating is the result of many complex and interacting factors

- see more clearly how our overeating works, including all the intended and unintended consequences of overeating

- recognise that although it is not our fault that we overeat (because we are 'set up' for it in so many ways), it is our responsibility to resolve it

- think carefully, from an encouraging and supportive perspective, about how to move forward to being the kind of person we want to be and coping with things in our lives in a way that we're happy with

- acknowledge the need for compassion, understanding and encouragement on our journey towards becoming that person

- think about and plan which aspects of our overeating to work on first

- see if the work we are doing is successfully tackling the factors that trigger our overeating and to keep it going.

Always keep in mind that this is a *compassionate* formulation, developed from within a compassionate mindset – that is, from a genuine intention and desire to understand and care for ourselves. It is not another tool with which to beat ourselves up for failure or non-achievement! In this chapter we have explored how Alison's personal history influenced the way she ate. In the next chapter we will explore a number of ways you can do this too.

My personal reflections on Chapter 10

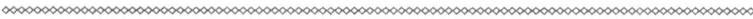

You might find it helpful to write down your key personal learning points from this chapter.

- What was it like to think about how your threat, drive and soothing systems influence your eating?

- Has this given you any ideas for what you might do differently or need to work on, when these systems come online?

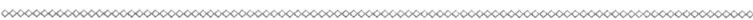

SUMMARY

In this chapter, we have worked on developing your personal formulation for overeating. At this stage we have focused on a 'here and now' formulation – looking at how threat, drive and soothing systems impact on your relationship with eating, and how you might use food to help you cope with your emotions. This can have intended consequences that help you feel less threatened, more excited or calmer, but may also have unintended consequences that can keep you trapped in unhelpful cycles, leaving you very critical of yourself and feeling hopeless. Please remember that none of this is your fault, it is the consequence of our tricky brains and bodies. The good news is that understanding these patterns is the first step to making positive changes. Your diary can be a valuable way of recording your 'here and now' relationship with eating. It can help you to identify a wide range of influences on your eating and will be the basis for your plan to overcome overeating, which we will explore in the final chapters of this book.

In the next chapter we will explore how our culture and personal history can significantly impact the development of our threat system, as well as how our past can influence our eating now. I will help you to pull all this together to develop a detailed compassionate formulation like we saw in Alison's example.

11 Putting it all together – a compassionate formulation for your overeating

Compassionate formulation: three levels

One way to make it easier to make sense of overeating patterns is to break them down into more manageable chunks (levels). In this chapter, we will explore several different ways to do this.

Level 1 compassionate formulations

This level helps us to understand which emotional regulation system (threat, drive or soothing) we are currently in and how this links with our eating. This requires us to tolerate our emotional states long enough to notice our thoughts and feelings, without trying to turn them off immediately. This can be challenging, and you will require the skills you have learned so far in this book to help you. At this stage we are not focusing on *why* we are in a particular emotional system; we simply need to notice it and think about whether we are likely to use overeating to cope. Your diary (Chapter 9) can help you to record which of the 'three systems' you were in when you overate. It may be that you rapidly jump between systems – for example, comfort eating to deal with anxiety (threat) then jumping to excitement linked to planning your new diet (drive). This is very common, so your level 1 formulation may need to include different systems that run at the same time or very close together – yet another example of how tricky our minds can be! This level of formulation can be very helpful if we find it difficult to recall our personal histories or identify specific triggers to our emotional states.

In Chapter 10, we looked at this in some detail. The first seven questions on Worksheet 11, 'How my eating works now' (page 278), can all help you explore your level 1 formulation. You might want to answer the questions over several weeks to explore the different ways your three systems interact with your eating (and each other).

How my eating works now (a reminder):

1. Am I at greater risk of overeating when my threat system comes online?

2. What types of threat emotions are most likely to trigger my overeating?

3. Are there any other threats that I pay attention to once my threat system is active?

4. How does eating help me to cope when my threat system is switched on?

5. Does eating help me to feel soothed?

6. Does eating help me turn off or tone down my threat system?

7. Does eating activate my drive system?

Drawing your three circles: a visual way to do your level 1 formulation

This is another way to make sense of your mind and how different systems can link to eating and help you to manage your thoughts and feelings more generally. This is something I often use with clients if they prefer to work visually. It is also an exercise my clients often use long after they have found a better relationship with food and eating, either as a daily, weekly or monthly check-in with themselves to help them to manage life's challenges and enhance their wellbeing.

We will break this down into a series of steps, to get a sense of how your three systems are operating and what you might deliberately do to change your motivational and emotional state.

As you may recall from Chapter 10, in a compassion focused approach we are interested in three main systems:

1. the threat system, which is mainly about helping to stop us doing, or get us away from, things that we believe are unpleasant or dangerous to us; the main emotions in this system include fear/anxiety, anger and disgust

2. the drive system, which is concerned with helping us reach specific goals; the main emotions in this system are excitement, celebration and pride

3. the affiliative contentment/soothing system, which focuses on making us feel calm and cared for.

It can be helpful to colour-code these, particularly when we are drawing them out. The usual coding is red for threat, blue for drive and green for soothing, but you can use any colours you want as long as you use the same ones every time.

For the next four exercises you will need four sheets of A4 paper, three coloured pencils and about thirty minutes.

Exercise 11.1: Drawing my three circles

To start with, you will draw the relative size of your three circles. You need to fit all three on one side of A4, and to leave some space between each circle because, towards the end of the exercise, you may need to draw arrows connecting them. We are going to start with what you think the relative size of each circle is today. The circles are a bit like balloons, they will inflate and deflate depending on your circumstances, relationships, mood, health and so on, and they can change minute by minute, hour by hour, day by day or week to week. The key to the exercise is to use the drawing to have sense of where you are at in the current moment. You can explore why they might be the way they are when we look at level 2 and level 3 formulations later in the chapter. For now, we are just looking at how you experience them in the present moment, to give you an idea if you need to inflate of deflate any. Please remember that the drawings are only meant to represent how you experience each circle, don't worry too much about exact sizes, just use the exercise to reflect on your felt sense of your circles. You can see an example in Figure 11.1.

Figure 11.1 Relative sizes of the three circles – an example

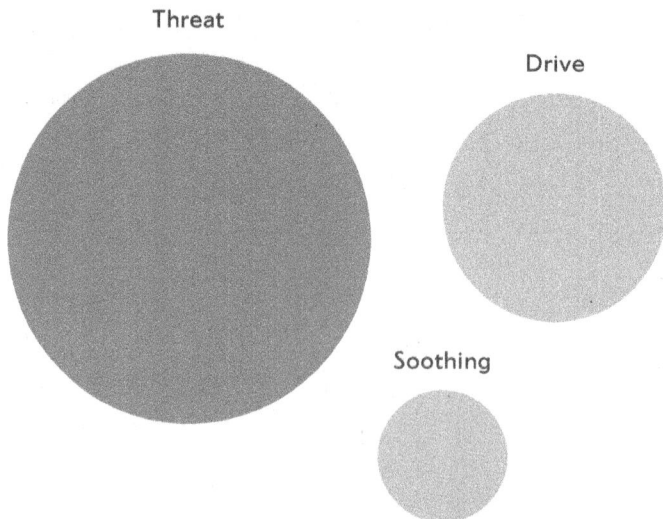

What do you notice about Figure 11.1? It looks as if threat is in the driving seat! The person who drew this does have access to all three circles. However, sometimes this is not the case if people find it difficult to have any sense of fun or achievement (low or no drive) or find it very difficult to be soothed. If we wanted to help this person find a better balance between their circles, we might want to help them understand, and ideally reduce, their threat system, and increase the things they do to turn on, or grow, their drive and soothing systems.

Once you have drawn your own circles, you may decide that you need to inflate or deflate them. The next exercises can help you explore ways to do this.

You will need your remaining three sheets of A4 paper. However, this time you will fill each one with a circle to represent either threat, drive or soothing. Most people start with the threat circle, but if this is too difficult for you, then start with either drive or soothing. Don't worry if the circles are not very big (as in Figure 11.1), all we are going to do is to find out what helps you experience drive or soothing.

Exercise 11.2: Drawing the drive system

Let's start with drive. In Figure 11.2 you can see, in the form of a pie chart, the types of things this person does to get a sense of achievement and to have fun.

Figure 11.2 Drive system pie chart

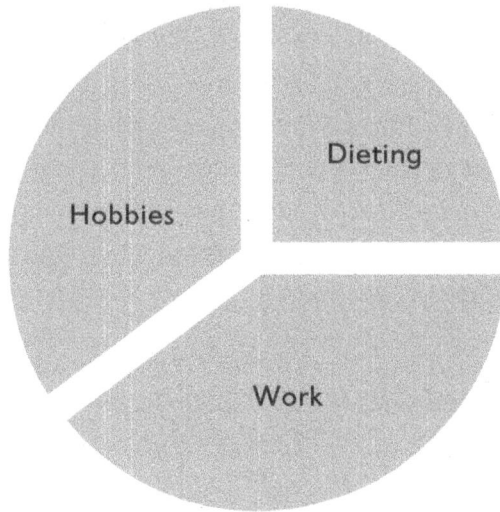

When we explore this drive pie chart it is important to note that this person gets a lot of their sense of achievement from dieting – this could be a problem if they are working on changing their eating and letting go of a dieting mindset. In this case they will need to find other ways to increase their joy from the drive system – perhaps by increasing the time spent doing their current hobbies, or finding new things to help them feel a sense of achievement (for example, from looking after their body and wellbeing).

We can always break this down more – for example, drawing a pie chart specifically of what hobbies or other things help this person to increase their drive. This understanding can then be used to develop an action plan, and maybe to drop activities that they think they *should* be enjoying but actually make them feel worse (like an old hobby that is now boring or a chore), or that give them a buzz but maybe have unintended side effects (for example, dieting). You can now try to draw your own drive chart.

Exercise 11.3: Drawing the soothing system

Next, you can draw the soothing system. Often this is relatively small to begin with and will need building up. Again, please draw a circle to fill a sheet of A4, as this will make it a bit easier to see the things you do alone, or with other people, that help you feel calm and content. It is OK if there is an overlap with things you do in your drive system (for example, a hobby you do alone or with friends). You can then put these into a pie chart. See Figure 11.3 for what this might look like.

Figure 11.3 Soothing system pie chart

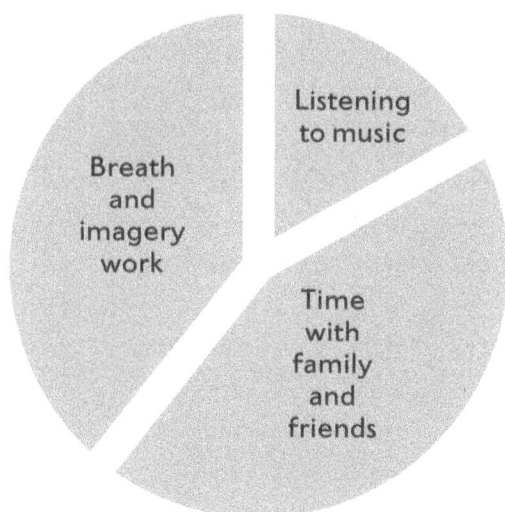

Figure 11.3 shows how some of the skills you are learning in this book (such as breath work or imagery) may become part of how you turn on your soothing system. It also shows the importance of spending time with family and friends, or solitary activities such as listening to music. As we have seen, it is important to have a variety of soothing activities, and to spend time actively fostering this system. Sadly, not everyone has family or friends they can talk to whenever they need, hence learning and practising ways

to soothe ourselves. When we are in a high threat state we often pull away from others, and it can be helpful to remind ourselves to connect with people who can help us, if we are fortunate enough to have them in our lives. If not, we may need to actively work on seeking out opportunities to build mutually supportive social connections, or connections with voluntary or professional support networks.

Exercise 11.4: Drawing the threat system

This is a slightly different exercise, as you are not looking at the things you do to create an emotional state (excitement or calm contentment). Instead, you are trying to map out different emotions which you experience in your threat system. We will concentrate on just three – anxiety, anger and disgust – mainly to make it easier for us to draw! You may of course have other emotions in this circle, such as envy, jealously, sadness or grief. The key is to put in the ones that you find difficult to experience and manage.

Figure 11.4 Threat system pie chart

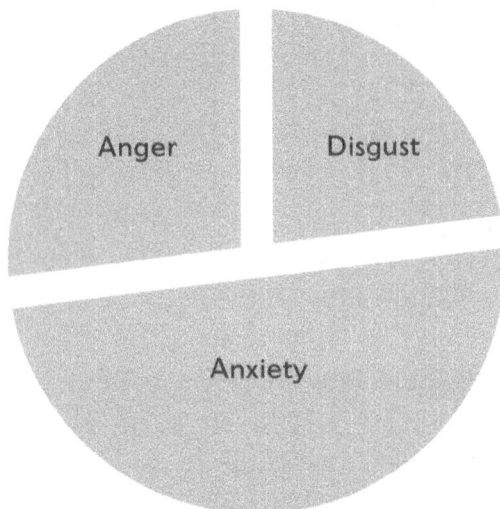

We can make sense of this system by taking each part and exploring it in more detail. You might find the following questions helpful.

1. Is my anger, anxiety or disgust focused on me or others, or both?

We may find that most of our anger is directed at ourselves, but very little at others, even if our compassionate mind would see them as mean or cruel to us. If this is the case, we might need to work on self-criticism and being compassionately assertive with people who accidentally or deliberately hurt us.

It may be that most of our anxiety is focused on people being critical or rejecting of us; if so, we may need to work on the social aspects of our anxiety. Or it may be that we are more anxious about our health, and this may become an issue we need to address. Perhaps our feelings of disgust are linked to our needs to eat or body shape, or we find that we become disgusted by others' shape or eating. This deeper analysis can help us work out the themes that are triggering for us, and help us to decide what we want to focus a more detailed formulation (level 2 or 3) on later, particularly if the way we cope with these issues impacts on our relationship with food, our body, relationships or overall wellbeing.

2. How does the threat system regulate itself?

You might notice that when your angry mind starts to come online (perhaps because other people are being mean to you), the anxious part of your threat system turns up to dampen this down. This can often be the case if we are taught that anger is bad or will lead to violence. It may be that when your anxious mind comes online, your angry mind becomes hostile and critical towards you for feeling scared. Or that when you feel disgust with yourself, perhaps because of the way you eat, your angry and anxious minds combine to shut this down (by focusing on the fear of rejection from others and angrily labelling you as weak and out of control). As painful as this can be, it may help you by moving your mind away from self-disgust.

These threat system jumps can often happen very fast and are our brain's way of trying to protect us from powerful emotions. Recognising how our brain does this can focus our compassion-ate mind on what we really need help with (for example, our feelings of disgust about eating). You can draw these connections between the parts of your threat system if this helps you to make sense of it. Further down the line your compassionate mind will help you accept and then work on these links (or even loops) without blaming you for them.

3. Does our drive or soothing system help regulate specific aspects of our threat system?

To answer this question, we can look for links between our threat system themes and the way we usually make them more toler-able via the things we do in our drive or soothing system. For example, does spending time doing a hobby shift our attention from feelings of anger at other people; does focusing on planning a diet help settle our feelings of disgust about our body?

Of course, this does not resolve the issues that triggered our threat system, and these themes often re-emerge when we stop doing things in our drive system, but it can give us some respite.

Similar patterns might occur when our soothing system comes online – for example, spending time focusing on soothing imagery may settle our feelings of anxiety, or being with people who care about us may help us feel less fearful of other people's negative judgements about our body.

As we become aware of these connections, and the triggers and themes of our threat system, it can be easier to plan soothing or drive system responses that we can use when our threat system comes online or might come online. With clients, I prefer to focus on soothing system responses, as these can help calm us enough to use our compassionate mind to work out why we are in threat, to listen to the wisdom of the threat system (for example, if it comes online because someone has been mean to us) and to find compassionate solutions. Of course, this does not mean that we are wrong to feel upset, hurt and angry if people are mean to us. Our compassionate mind will acknowledge and care for us during this painful period. It will help us work out, and have the courage to adopt, new ways of dealing with this that don't involve being mean to ourselves for being upset or using coping strategies (often automatically) that may have longer-term side effects (such as overeating).

Level 2 compassionate formulations

Sometimes level 1 formulations can be enough for you to recognise you are in a system (e.g. threat) and choose to stop overeating and do something else to help you instead. However, sometimes we can get stuck in loops that are difficult to break free from. Our tricky brain often does not want us to break out of the loop, because it thinks it is the best way to help us. It might tell us, 'So what – you can eat when you're anxious or sad and it won't harm you.' It is only doing this because it wants things to be better for us, but this can blind us to understanding what issues we actually need help with and to the unintended consequences. Sometimes we don't notice these consequences until after an overeating episode and then can beat ourselves up about them.

In level 2 we are interested in what things immediately trigger our three systems and shift us into a mindset associated with overeating. Your diary can be really helpful here. We are also interested in what we do or think to help us manage the emotions that are linked to overeating. We can think about this as the *intended consequences* of our responses. We need to be a little careful here – *intended consequences* do not mean we always plan things out in advance or are fully aware of why we react in the way we do and the impact this has on us or others. They are simply how we manage in the moment, often based on previous learning, habit or our brain's best guess about what will work to help us deal with difficult situations or feelings, or to help us feel good. If they do work, even just in the short term, we are likely to stick to them. The key here is to understand connections, not to beat ourselves up for finding ways to cope with life.

The final step of a level 2 formulation is to understand the *unintended consequences* of our responses – the side effects of coping in the way we do. This is the area where I find people can become the most self-critical. It is important to remember that we are usually unaware of the side effects (for better or worse) of our actions. For example, I never knew that my first training placement with Professor Gilbert thirty years ago would lead to me writing this book! Compassionately noticing our unintended consequences can help us explore whether we want to keep responding in the way we do to things (e.g. comfort eating when we are upset) and to manage the side effects of this way of coping (e.g. gaining weight) in new ways.

The last two questions on Worksheet 11, 'How my eating works now' (page 278), can help you explore this. They are:

8. What do I hope that eating will make me feel (the intended consequence of eating)?

9. What are the unintended consequences of overeating?

It is likely that overeating helps or has helped you in a variety of ways, either in the past or right now, and you may have to spend some time unpacking the answers to these two questions. If overeating no longer helps you manage difficulties, it is possible that it has now become a habit, but this can still be difficult to break, and beating yourself up about it just adds insult to injury.

Level 3 compassionate formulations

Level 1 and 2 formulations tend to look at 'how' questions. For example, *how* do I eat when I am angry, *how* does this help me in the short term, *how* does it create longer-term problems for me? Level 3 formulations look at 'why' questions. For example, *why* do I eat the way I do, *why* am I so self-critical? This can be the most difficult level of formulation, as it often means looking to our past to understand our thoughts, feelings and actions in the present, or our fears and hopes for the future.

We will now look at ways you can make sense of your history, and how this links to key threats, safety strategies, and the intended and unintended consequences that can create the vicious feedback loops that make it so difficult to stop overeating.

Making sense of your history

This can be quite difficult, as we may not have many easily accessible memories of our early years, and our minds can actually help us to not think about difficult events in our lives. However, doing this can be helpful to us in making sense of things, not beating ourselves up for how we are, and finding new solutions to life's challenges that don't involve overeating. Our history includes the culture we grew up in or live in now, our personal experiences of growing up (e.g. at school) and our experiences (for better or worse) with people (including family and friends).

I think it is often easier to start by examining cultural influences. One way to do this is to spend some time looking at how types of food and eating (or not eating) are sold to us in mainstream or social media. For example, you can look at how food is promoted as a treat after having a bad day or observe how many adverts there are for diets. These influences can be very hard to resist, and of course we do not want to remove the joy we get from eating, but it can be helpful to think about other ways you can experience pleasure and comfort or manage difficult emotions and situations.

Making sense of our personal history can be challenging. Sometimes it can help to develop a timeline of events and link this to times when overeating became more important or frequent in your life. As always, take this at a pace you feel you can manage, and always look at your past from the perspective of your compassionate mind. Please remember, you did not choose the events life sent your way, and using food to help yourself is likely to be one of the few ways you could cope at the time.

An eating timeline

Below you will find an example of a timeline. As you will see, there are two parts to this. The first identifies important events in a person's life. These experiences may have led to comfort eating, eating to punish yourself, restricting eating, bingeing, etc.

Some of the events that people find difficult to manage include:

- losses

- bereavements

- moving home, work or schools – especially those situations that require us to make new friends

- difficult relationships and interpersonal conflicts

- setbacks that give us feelings of disappointment or of being a failure

- emotionally, physically or sexually abusive experiences.

Sometimes more positive experiences can also lead to overeating episodes, as we may associate eating with celebrations or being more relaxed. It is important to write down both kinds of events in your timeline.

Eating patterns may also be associated with periods of deliberate or accidental weight loss. So, again, it is important to note the times you have dieted and lost or gained weight. If you have lost weight, it can also be helpful to understand *how* or *why* this happened – for example, because you were ill or taking medication. Some people will not have specific events that have triggered periods of overeating. It may be more about the way we have grown up learning to eat.

In Figure 11.5 you will find a copy of David's timeline. We will spend some time in the next section using David's example as a way of learning to fill in and interpret your own timeline.

Figure 11.5 David's eating timeline

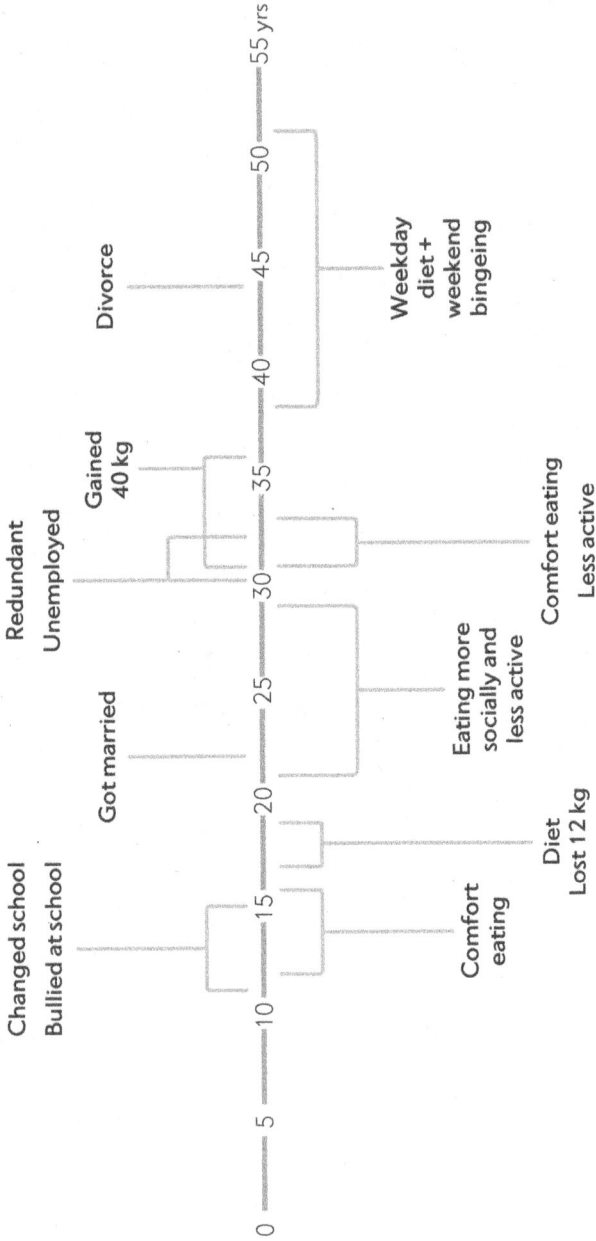

Figure 11.5 David's eating timeline

Using a timeline: what David learned

Eating and weight loss history

David was fifty-three when he completed his timeline. He remembered struggling with eating for most of his life. He believed this was because he was greedy or had poor self-control. He found it difficult to remember when and how his difficulties with eating began. I suggested that he complete a timeline in several phases. First, just to write down the times in his life when he had noticed changes in his weight, either significantly gaining or losing weight. Most people's weight does tend to fluctuate a bit, so we focused on times when he had changed by more than half a stone (3 kg) and when the change had lasted for more than three months. I then asked him to note down the times he had dieted, how long for, and how much his weight had changed from the start of the diet to six months after he had finished. Next, he noted when his 'overeating mind' was active. Finally, I asked David to write down the important events in his life, even if he did not think that they had had an impact on his eating. This included unpleasant experiences, but also things that he found more positive.

We then put all four timelines together. David came to several conclusions about the connections between the events in his life and his eating patterns. Understandably he had tried not to think about the unpleasant experiences of being bullied, but he recalled being very unhappy, with no one to talk to at that time in his life. He also remembered that he would hide away in the local shop at school lunchtimes and eat sweets and biscuits. The local shopkeeper was very kind and would give him sweets while he waited, and he learned to associate food with being cared for and safe. However, he also felt bad about gaining weight so would become very self-critical if he felt he had overeaten.

David recognised that dieting had made him feel better about himself, helping him feel in control and more confident. However, he also noticed that when he was happier (e.g. when he met and married his wife, and when things were going well at work) he was more relaxed around eating, he took more joy in food and in eating socially. His weight was stable at this time.

David's biggest weight change and most severe episodes of binge-eating followed being made redundant and being unemployed for about eighteen months. He described this as a very dark time. It became clear that he was actually quite depressed, as many people can be who are made redundant. David's weight gain worried him and so he began a period of dieting during the week, followed by bingeing at weekends, but he had maintained the weight gain, despite his pattern of dieting in the week. Interestingly, David also noticed that his divorce had relatively little effect on his eating or his weight.

David was able to complete his timeline but remained very critical of his eating. So, I asked him to look at the timeline from the perspective of his compassionate mind and as if it belonged to someone he cared about. This helped him gain a bit of distance from the way he normally thought about himself (as lazy and greedy). David was able to acknowledge that if these events had happened to someone else, he could accept that there was a connection between events in their life and their eating patterns, and he became more compassionately motivated to be less self-critical of his eating and able to disconnect eating from managing life events and emotions. He also recognised that, if he was not in a high state of threat, he could enjoy eating more and eat socially without it leading to overeating episodes.

Key steps to developing your own timeline

Before you begin to write your own timeline, it is helpful to activate your compassionate mind. Begin by bringing your soothing system online. When you are ready, also bring your compassionate image online. You can then start to reflect on your past from the perspective of your compassionate image. If you find you become self-critical as you write your timeline, that is perfectly normal, as we all have a tendency to blame ourselves for the things that happen to us. Just pause, re-engage your soothing system and compassionate image, then spend a little time thinking about what feelings your self-critical mindset is helping you to manage. You may then need to spend some time being self-compassionate with these difficult feelings. Your compassionate mind may help you to do this by understanding your need to tolerate these feelings for a short time, while you understand your past. It will also know how much of this you can take, and to offer you soothing activities or distractions if these feelings become too much to bear. In this case you may want to stop the exercise for a while and come back to it when you feel ready. It can also be helpful to give yourself a time limit for working on your timeline, perhaps for five to ten minutes to begin with, and to plan to have something soothing or distracting to do when you finish. Please remember that the aim is to develop your own understandings of your history, not to see how much pain you can tolerate!

So let us think about starting to write down your timeline. You can begin at the present day or from when you were born. It can be easier to make sense of time by going in five-year steps or by picking significant changes in your life, like starting school, your first job, first relationship, etc. It really doesn't matter which units of time you use, as long as it makes sense to you. It is likely that you may not remember all of the things that have led to overeating, particularly if this began in early life. This is fine; remember this is one way of helping you make sense of your history, which in turn can help you towards developing a compassionate understanding of your relationship with food in the past.

Don't worry if you find this difficult; just do the best you can. Your timeline will never be perfect as none of us has a perfect recall of all the things that have happened to us! The main aim is to help you make connections between events in your life and overeating.

To summarise, the key steps are:

- Write down the times in your life when you noticed gaining weight by more than half a stone and for more than three months.

- Write down when you have dieted, and for how long, and how much your weight changed from the start of the diet to six months after you had finished.

- Write down the times when your overeating mindsets (e.g. 'comfort food' or 'dieting mind') were active for more than a month at a time.

- Write down the important events in your life, even if you do not think that they had an impact on your eating. This includes unpleasant experiences and more positive ones.

- Put these timelines together and look for any connections. It can help to imagine that you are spotting connections for someone else.

In Worksheet 12 I have provided a timeline that you could use to help you make sense of your overeating. You can use this as a template or, alternatively, you can develop your own. Please feel free to use this as a model, but, as we have seen from David's example, it may be easier to break this down into chunks before putting all of the information together.

Worksheet 12: My overeating timeline

Important life events

Weight gain history

0 ——— 5 ——— 10 ——— 15 ——— 20 ——— 25 ——— 30 ——— 35 ——— 40 ——— 45 ——— 50 ——— 55 ——— 60 ——— 65 yrs

Overeating

Dieting and weight-loss history

Once you have completed your timeline you may have some more ideas about the way in which your past has influenced your relationship with eating. Often, reminders of these events, or the feelings they are linked to, can be current triggers to overeating or a negative relationship with food.

When you have finished your timeline, you may also wish to think about how your cultural and personal history have combined to influence your relationship with eating. You can explore these using the questions in Exercise 11.5.

Exercise 11.5: Links between my culture and history and their influences on my eating and relationship with myself

- How does the culture I live in influence my relationship with eating?

- What were the important personal experiences that influenced my relationship with eating (e.g. 'food as fun' or a dieting mindset)?

- What experiences in my past have influenced the way I treat myself now (e.g. self-critically)?

You might then spend some time thinking about and writing down your answers to the following questions.

- What are my key learning points from doing a timeline?

- What compassionate things would I want to say to someone I cared about who had had the experiences I had? Would I blame them for their struggles with food and eating?

Putting it all together: level 3 compassionate formulations

The final exercises in this chapter help you put together all the information you have gathered so far to develop a level 3 compassionate formulation of your eating. You can use the same exercises to work out other things about yourself – for example, self-criticism, or your relationship with your body. But for now, we are going to focus on your relationship with food and eating. This is the same method we used to work out Alison's relationship with eating in Chapter 10 (pages 270–92). You might want to reread that section now to remind yourself of the process.

As for every other exercise we do, please turn on your soothing system and then engage your compassionate mind to do each exercise. It is unlikely you will do this all in one go. Take your time and do as much, or as little, as your compassionate mind thinks you can. If you notice you become self-critical, just stop, do something soothing and distracting, and come back to it when you are in your compassionate mind. It is likely there are multiple answers to each of the questions. This is because our tricky minds often have a lot going on in them and tend to use a single solution (such as overeating) to manage multiple difficulties. If this is the case then don't worry, you will need to look for a compassionate solution for each element of the puzzle so that overeating is no longer the best solution. This can take a while, but it will give you a longer-term way of managing life's challenges, and will lead to a better relationship with food, eating and yourself.

Exercise 11.6: Drawing up a level 3 compassionate formulation for my eating

1. What are my key threats?

This is where you identify the things that trigger your threat system. Remember, these may involve a range of different emotions – for example, sadness, anger, disgust or grief. You may find it helpful to use the notes you have made about your timeline and from your eating diary to identify times when you have had to deal with events and emotions that you have found difficult. You can then look for patterns. Are there any themes that you have found trigger your threat system (e.g. arguments with other people, feeling lonely, worrying whether people like you)?

Now try to list:

My key threats linked to overeating

1.

2.

3.

and any others . . .

The next section looks at past influences. Some of these will be linked to your personal experiences, some to noticing the lives of others, some to your culture, and some will be a combination of these influences.

Now try to list:

The past influences on my key threats

1.

2.

3.

and any others . . .

The current triggers to my key threats

1.

2.

3.

and any others . . .

2. What are my safety strategies?

These are the things that you do, feel or think to help you manage your key threats. Alison's example mainly explored her behavioural safety strategies (e.g. trying to please others, comfort eating and dieting). Other strategies can include thoughts that protect you from powerful emotions, such as not allowing yourself to get close to others, or always blaming yourself when things go wrong. They can also include habitual emotional reactions, such as disgust, to keep us away from things we find threatening.

If you find it difficult to identify these thoughts and emotions, it may be helpful to consider what other people might notice that you do to protect yourself; perhaps talk this over with someone you trust.

Now try to list:

My safety strategies

1.

2.

3.

and any others . . .

3. What are the intended consequences of my safety strategies?

We may use our safety strategies in a very deliberate way, or we may find that they have become something of a habit, with their original purpose lost.

Knowing what you aim to achieve or avoid by using a particular safety strategy makes it easier to start thinking about alternative ways to cope with the problem. However, sometimes you may need to give up the strategy for a short time before you become aware of the role eating has played and are able to start considering other ways to manage.

You might find that working on your key threats individually, linking each of them to a safety strategy (or several), helps you to work out what the intended consequences of each of your strategies are.

Now try to list:

The intended consequences for each of my safety strategies

1.

2.

3.

and any others . . .

4. What are the unintended consequences of my safety strategies?

We have now seen that some of our strategies have unintended consequences that can lead to further difficulties. It can be helpful to work on each strategy separately, using your personal history, diaries, your own wisdom and the helpful observations of others, to work out the unintended consequences of your own safety strategies.

Now try to list:

The unintended consequences of my safety strategies

1.

2.

3.

and any others . . .

Finally, you can explore whether these unintended consequences actually increase the level of threat you feel or encourage you to intensify your safety strategies.

Once you have completed your formulation, you are then in a position to start developing alternative strategies to manage your threat system. Your new understanding of your relationship with eating will help you to predict the types of problem that you will need help with, and the possible unintended consequences of changing your relationship with food. In the next chapter we will explore how we can use this new understanding to motivate you to make changes in your eating.

My personal reflections on Chapter 11

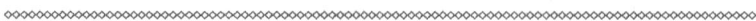

You might find it helpful to write down your key personal learning points from this chapter.

- What was it like to develop a level 3 compassionate formulation for your relationship with food and eating?

- Has this given you any ideas for what you might do differently or need to work on?

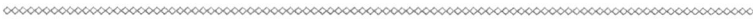

SUMMARY

In this chapter, we worked though the steps to developing your personal level 3 compassionate formulation for your relationship with food and eating. This relies, to some extent, on your own recollections of your personal history. If this is difficult, you might want to talk to someone who knows you well, and you can trust, to help make sense of your history. Please don't worry if you cannot remember things. Our minds often try to forget the most painful events in our lives, or only remember the difficult, rather than joyful, experiences we have. Both are ways our brains have evolved to protect us. If thinking about the past is too difficult or painful then you can stay with a level 1 (three circles) formulation or a level 2 formulation – focusing your attention on times when your threat system is triggered and how you cope.

Hopefully these exercises have given you an idea of the things you may want to work on to make overeating less necessary to help you with difficult emotions or experiences, or to find comfort and pleasure.

Understanding ourselves better is a great first step. However, making changes requires motivation, dedication and the ability to 'bounce back' from setbacks. We will explore these themes in Chapter 12.

12 Compassionately motivating yourself to change

In this chapter, we will explore a way of understanding how the process of changing our behaviour, thoughts and feelings works. If you are reading this book, it is likely that you are at least considering changing your eating and relationship with food. Indeed, you may well have tried to do this in the past. As we shall see, change can be difficult, and sometimes we can feel like we are taking one step forward and two back. It is really easy to get disheartened and give up, or blame ourselves for our 'weakness'. This chapter will help you understand why 'failure' and setbacks are an inevitable part of the process of change. We will explore how to make the most of these setbacks and address overeating for good.

This chapter is all about preparing you to make changes. By the end you will have the tools to keep you motivated and be able to understand how and why setbacks take place and to respond to them compassionately.

The seven stages of change

Psychologists are very interested in how people change. The good news is that people can and do change, and we have much better ideas about how to make this happen than we used to. Two pioneers in this field, James Prochaska and Carlo DiClemente, were particularly interested in helping people give up physically and psychologically addictive behaviour, such as smoking and alcohol misuse, and they worked out a model of how change happens that has now been widely applied to a range of difficulties, including eating problems. Many people I have worked with have found this useful in helping them to understand where they are in relation to the stages of change, and to work out how to move towards permanently overcoming overeating.

Prochaska and DiClemente identified seven stages in the change process, from not thinking about change to changing for good. Let's take a look at how these stages may work.

Pre-contemplation

In this stage, we are not trying to address our overeating. We are likely to be caught up in eating mindsets (e.g. comfort eating, dieting, food as fun or food as punishment). We may become quite defensive or dismissive if people talk to us about our overeating, express concern or try to make us change our relationship with food.

Contemplation

Here we are likely to be thinking about or discussing our overeating. For example, you may have been in this stage when you were reading the early chapters of this book. This stage can often be quite distressing, as we think about the impact that overeating has had on us and the various reasons we have needed overeating to help us cope with our situation or emotions. This is a stage that can often be difficult to tolerate, and people often move back into pre-contemplation to avoid this distress. If we are going to beat overeating (or any other problem in our lives, for that matter) it is really important to remember that this suffering is a purposeful step on the journey of change. It is part of the 'engagement with suffering' aspect of compassion and the process of formulation that we looked at in chapters 10 and 11. As we noted, we do not need to beat ourselves up for having overeaten in the past; this was the result of your experiences, combined with a tricky brain and body.

Preparation

This is a stage in which we are planning to make change and getting ready to move forward. The more time we put into this stage, the better chance we have of success. Sometimes we can feel in a rush to do something about our difficulties; this is understandable but can lead to unintended consequences that can accidentally sabotage things later on. The work you have done in completing your compassionate formulation and eating diaries is part of this stage.

Your formulations should help you manage some of the unintended consequences of change, but it is important to remember that there is no such thing as 'perfect preparation'. This stage can sometimes feel rather overwhelming, as we notice the many things that overeating may have helped us with. So, as part of preparing for change (and the distress it may bring with it for a time), we need to prepare for making small and achievable changes, and to be aware that sometimes change will have unintended consequences or help you to learn something new about yourself that will need to be incorporated as you revise your formulations and action plans.

Action

In this stage, which we will cover in the next four chapters of the book, we are putting our plans into action. This is often hard work and can be quite frustrating, but it can also be very satisfying and empowering to learn new ways to manage life's challenges. Change can be quite a slow process, and there can be unintended consequences or obstacles, which may seem disheartening at the time. To have the best chance of coping with these, it is really important to have reasons for making this change that are important to you, and ideally also to have support from others. This does not mean that we can't change if we don't have external support. For example, developing a compassionate relationship with yourself and using compassionate mind exercises (e.g. 'me at my best' or compassionate companion) can give you someone in your corner cheering you on and commiserating when things get tough.

Maintenance

In this stage, we tend to find that the changes we have made have become easier to manage and gradually become positive habits. However, sometimes this can lull us into thinking that our old coping styles are changed for good. It can be relatively easy to forget the things that are helping us to address overeating, and the issues that triggered it, and to see any setback as a sign that the work we did before was wasted, or that we are weak in some way.

Lapses

It's almost inevitable that we will have a 'lapse' or setback at some point. Lapses are more likely to be triggered when our new coping strategies are becoming established. However, they can also occur when we face new or unfamiliar situations. For example, we may have managed to reduce our overeating at home very well, but then go on holiday with friends who encourage us to overeat. Lapses can also occur when we try to push changes too fast – for example, moving quickly from establishing a structured approach to managing our eating to learning to rely on our hunger and satiety system to inform us when we are full. The key thing here is to have a plan for managing lapses; one that sees them as part of a normal learning curve, rather than as taking you back to square one.

It is likely that we will sometimes move from a lapse back into a period of pre-contemplation, or even into a prolonged period of overeating. Don't worry – we all go through these times when we are making changes. The key is to learn from our lapses and, when we are ready, to move on to the next phase of the process of change. With practice, this process of recovery becomes quicker each time, and indeed you may even learn to welcome the occasional lapse to remind you that you do have the skill and courage to overcome setbacks. Many people find that they feel better about themselves for knowing that they have the strength to do this.

Termination

At this point, we find that our new strategies have stood the test of time. We have learned to manage and overcome the obstacles to changing our eating habits.

Why think about the process of change?

The key reasons for thinking about this process are to:

- remind us that we are only human, that change takes time, and that we will all have setbacks

- help us recognise what stage we are in and to work with

rather than against it – for example, it is OK to think about changing (contemplation) for some time before taking action, but we may need to plan to support ourselves through any distress this may cause us

- help us develop realistic expectations of the amount of time and energy we may need to devote to making changes

- develop a sense that facing obstacles and making mistakes is normal and OK.

If we are in the *contemplation* stage, we may need to spend more time thinking about the potential benefits of change, as well as the costs, before we are ready to move on.

If we are in the *preparation* stage, we may need to think about our plans for addressing overeating: how we can develop small and achievable targets that will help us towards our goals; any potential obstacles that we're aware of; the support we might need and where we might get it from; and the skills we may need to develop to help us put our plans into action.

If we are in the *action* phase, we may need to think about the amount of time and energy we can devote to changing, how we will keep ourselves motivated and how we will manage lapses.

In the *maintenance* phase, we may need to work on recognising the changes we have made and encouraging ourselves to maintain them, reminding ourselves of the benefits of change, and again to think about how we manage lapses.

Compassionate motivation

As you may recall from Chapter 4, one of the key attributes of a compassionate mind is compassionate motivation. This comes from a deep caring for the wellbeing of ourselves and others that generates a decision and commitment to help care for and relieve suffering. Sometimes other mindsets can block us from alleviating our suffering or encourage us to use short-term solutions that can inadvertently lead to further distress in the long run. Compassionate motivation tends to take a longer-term view and is also interested in helping us with the unintended consequences of the ways we manage distress (such as overeating) and in caring for us as we make these changes.

When we bring this together with an understanding of the process of change, it can be very powerful in helping us remain motivated in our quest. It can also help us to understand and deal compassionately with the inevitable lapses and setbacks that will occur.

The exercises that follow are designed to help you explore and develop your motivation to change. Before you begin, set aside some time to bring your compassionate image into mind – either your compassionate self or your compassionate companion. When you are ready, imagine yourself as a deeply compassionate person who fully understands why we overeat – for reasons beyond our control – and why managing eating is hard.

Focus on a sense of warmth and kindness. Let your face settle into a compassionate expression. Imagine how you might speak to someone with gentle understanding and encouragement. What would your tone of voice and pace of speaking sound like?

If you prefer, you can imagine how your compassionate image/companion would motivate you to resolve overeating. In that case you would imagine their dedication to you, their wisdom, kindness and strength. Again, pay attention to imagining their tone of voice.

When you think you have created this mindset, at least to some extent, then you can begin the exercises. Try to spend a couple of minutes on each of the following exercises at first and write down whatever comes to mind. You can return to the exercises whenever you find any new things that can motivate you, or if you lose motivation to work on your overeating.

Exercise 12.1: What stage of change am I in and how can I move forward?

This first exercise helps us to think about what stage of change you are in at the moment. You can then use your compassionate mind to help you consider what would help you move into the next phase. Imagine considering and answering this question with kindness, openness, honesty and understanding.

Exercise 12.2: Recognising the benefits and costs of overeating

This exercise focuses on the contemplation and preparation stages of change. It will help you to identify reasons for changing your overeating, as well as the benefits of keeping overeating as part of your life.

Using all of the information you have gained from your timeline, formulations, eating diaries and any other sources, try to complete statements 1–7. Your personal compassionate formulation for overeating really comes into its own here. Remember, your compassionate mind knows that overeating may have been your best coping strategy in the past and it is not going to criticise you for it, only help you to take responsibility for seeking more, longer-term coping strategies in the future with fewer costs than overeating.

1.   My overeating helps me to manage:

2.   My overeating has had the following unintended consequences on my health:

3.   My overeating has had the following unintended consequences on my mood, thoughts and feelings:

4.   My overeating has had the following unintended consequences on my social life and relationships:

5.   My overeating has had the following unintended consequences on my occupational or academic life:

6.   In what ways would my life improve if I changed my eating and relationship with food?

7.   What would motivate me to give up overeating in the short term and the long term?

When you can answer the last two questions from a compassionate perspective, you are on the way to moving from the contemplation to the preparation stage.

It can be helpful to use your answers to these questions (we can call them your 'motivational lists') to provide a daily reminder of why you want to change. People I have worked with have found various ways to do this. These include:

- keeping them where you can easily see them (such as on the fridge door or the bathroom mirror, or even as a screen saver!)

- keeping them in a scrapbook to which you can add pictures, poems or letters that will help motivate you to change

- sharing your reasons for changing with someone who cares about you, and giving that person (or people) permission to remind you of why you want to change

- spending some time each day thinking about the reasons to change from the perspective of your compassionate mind.

Please remember that the things that will motivate you are personal to you. They may not always make logical sense, and they certainly won't be the same for everyone. Different things will motivate you at different times and, again, this is perfectly normal. The only real rule about motivation is that it must be compassionate. It must have our best interests at heart and should not involve bullying, cajoling or scaring us into change. This type of behaviour can work in the short term, but further down the line is only likely to result in us being more self-critical and miserable, or even rebelling against the very changes we want to encourage ourselves to make.

Improving your chances of success: planning for blocks to change

The final element of the preparation stage is to plan for potential blocks. Some of these will be specific to the exercises we will use to help us address overeating, and we will explore these as we introduce each activity. However, there may be more general blocks that we can address before you decide to begin changing your relationship with food and eating.

To address overeating, you will need to make time for yourself to work on the exercises in this book. This might be in short bursts (for example, spending a minute or so after each eating episode recording the details in your diary) or you may need to set aside an hour to plan your eating or write a compassionate letter. Finding this time can be very difficult, even if we really want to, so it is important that you see the work from the perspective of caring for yourself, and truly wanting to alleviate your suffering, rather than as something you have to criticise or bully yourself into doing!

Sometimes the commitments we have in our lives, or the people around us, can make it difficult to make the changes we want to. Again, it can be helpful to think about this in advance, especially if these obstacles are practical difficulties that we may need to find ways of working around. This can help give us the best chance of making permanent changes in the ways we eat.

You can use the next two exercises to think about any practical difficulties. Again, your compassionate mind's perspective can be helpful; it knows the difference between your fears of change and the real obstacles that we can all face. It will be wise enough to help you manage some of these practical problems without blaming you, or being angry with you, for the things that may slow you down as you overcome overeating. It may also be wise enough to know when you need help to address these obstacles, and to be brave enough to ask for and accept it.

Exercise 12.3: Identifying practical problems

Please list any practical problems that your compassionate mind can think of that may make it difficult for you to make time to change your overeating. For example, you may be just starting a new job or moving house, and this may leave you with very little time to do your compassion exercises or to plan your eating.

Exercise 12.4: Overcoming the practical problems

Now use your compassionate mind to help you plan how you might overcome some of these difficulties. So, you may decide to postpone starting your journey to eating compassionately until the house move is complete or you have settled into the new job. Or, knowing that the events are going to be stressful, you may decide to make some time to do your exercises and to eat regularly. Both are examples of a compassionate solution, as they recognise your limitations and support you to work with them, without criticising yourself for your solution!

Some things to try

While I can't know, of course, what your personal obstacles are, it might be helpful for you to consider how other people have managed to overcome some of the common obstacles you may well encounter.

Making time to plan

In the early stages of this process, you may need to learn to make time and space to eat and to reflect on your feelings before you change your eating – plan a few more breaks in the day, and try to create five minutes of 'me time' every couple of hours.

Focus your attention on changing

This can be difficult, too. There are so many other things that can pull us away, and it is very easy to fall back into old habits. Try to set up reminders of the times that you are going to eat, perhaps using an alarm on your phone.

Maintaining attention on the reasons and triggers for overeating

For example, you might put a note on your fridge that says, 'Do I really need to eat now?' Perhaps you can keep a notebook or send yourself a text message and save it for when you spot an urge to overeat, or when you have found a new way to cope.

Staying focused on why you are doing the work

Many people – perhaps 99 per cent of us – get disheartened when they're trying to change things, and it will be relatively easy to go back to not working on overeating, especially at first. Keep the motivational lists you made for Exercise 12.2 somewhere where you can look at them easily; maybe even do the exercise again when you notice that you want to give up or have had a lapse.

Another way to stay focused is to keep a scrapbook of the reasons why you want to change; this can include pictures, drawings, poetry, artwork – anything you like really that makes the reasons you want to change concrete and important to you. Focus on the kind of person you want to become and how eating well will make this more likely.

Focus on success

People who overeat tend to be quite self-critical and focus on their mistakes. It can help to get into the daily habit of writing down each small (or big) step you have taken in improving your eating and becoming more compassionate. You might want to keep this list in your scrapbook and look at it each morning when you get up.

Sometimes what we initially think are practical blocks (e.g. 'I don't have time') turn out to be linked to emotional blocks (e.g. 'I am worried what people will think of me if I make more time for myself') or to other worries about changing (e.g. 'How will I deal with my feelings if I can't use food when I am upset?'). It is absolutely normal to have both types of blocks. They key thing is to be compassionate about our limitations and with our concerns about changing.

It is helpful to be aware that the more blocks there are the longer it may take us to address overeating – but that does not mean we can't do it. The biggest single factor in predicting whether we will succeed is our desire for and commitment to change. That is why it's important to work out why you want to change your overeating and what will help keep you motivated when the going gets tough.

Getting support to help you address overeating

Overeating is something that many people feel ashamed of, and this can stop them from seeking appropriate support. This is something else that can undermine our chances of overcoming overeating or at least lengthen the time it takes. The next exercise involves using your compassionate mind to help you make a list of all the people who might support you. Your compassionate mind will be wise enough to know the difference between the fears that may stop you asking them to help and the reality of whether these people would genuinely want to help you. It is also wise to work out if the person is genuinely compassionate or has an ulterior, less caring motive. It is brave to risk letting people care, and to either allow them to help, or distance ourselves if they turn out to be unhelpful or even harmful to us. You might want to try by sharing a little of your difficulties at first to see how people respond, and if this works out well you can share a little more. Remember, it is up to your compassionate mind to decide if the person will be someone you turn to in the long term, and to decide the kinds of things you trust them to help you with.

Sometimes we can feel that people won't want to help, or if they do, they will see us as a burden. It is really important to remember that if people do care, they will want to help and if they help you, they will experience a sense of joy in being helpful and pride in you for changing. You might want to remember a time when you have helped them, or other people – how did this feel for you? When we can offer compassion, it is good for our brain and body, as well as potentially helpful to the person we offer it to. It helps us all to feel more connected and gives our lives greater meaning and purpose. Denying people who care about us the opportunity to help us (out of shame or fear) is not fair to them or us and is likely to make life a bit more miserable and difficult.

Your list could include family, friends, work colleagues, your doctor and perhaps a therapist. Of course, you may not wish to share everything about yourself with everyone on your list – in fact, some people can help without ever knowing you have a problem. For example, you may arrange to go out with someone because you enjoy their company and when you are with them you are less likely to overeat. There may be other people in your life who care for you and perhaps have a more compassionate view of you than you have of yourself. They can be really helpful in steering us away from the urge to beat ourselves up for the ways we eat, or drawing our attention to aspects of ourselves that our self-critical or tricky eating mindsets do not.

Before each exercise, bring your soothing system online and then move into your compassionate mind using the exercises that work best for you.

Exercise 12.5: Identifying sources of help

Use your compassionate mind to help you list the people who could help you work on overeating and what kind of help they may be able to give you (e.g. practical, emotional, distraction).

Person	What can they do to help me?

When you have developed your own plan for overcoming overeating, you may wish to talk with some of these people about how they can help. You may also wish to share this book with them and let them see your compassionate formulation, or the things you are doing to address overeating (such as your meal plan), so that they can support, encourage or even help you to make changes.

Compassionately managing setbacks

As we saw earlier, setbacks are to be expected when we try to change the way we eat (or anything else, for that matter). Again, we need to bring our compassionate mind to bear when we have a setback or lapse into overeating. If you were truly motivated to care for yourself, and to learn from and move forward from a setback, what kind of things would your compassionate mind say? Would it blame you, see you as inadequate or weak in some way? Or would it want to comfort and support you, to help you understand and learn from your setbacks?

Of course, in that moment of disappointment it may not be easy to maintain your compassionate mindset. So, it's a good idea to practise in advance how you might respond when that happens. To do this, first bring your compassionate mind online. Now imagine that you are supporting a friend who has tried to change their overeating but has had a setback – perhaps has lapsed back into overeating because they had gone to a party and got carried away with the joy of eating socially or had found out some upsetting news. How would you feel if you wanted them to eat well but had seen them struggle? What sort of thing would you like to say to them to help them be compassionately motivated to learn from the experience and to make a renewed commitment to work on their overeating?

When you have some idea of the things that your compassionate self would like to say to someone else, you could try writing a short compassionate letter to yourself that you can read when lapses occur. (We looked at writing compassionate letters in detail in Chapter 8.) This might include expressing your appreciation of your courage and wisdom for working on overeating, your sadness and your disappointment for the lapse, but also your support and encouragement for continuing the journey. You may also want to put down some ideas for the things that can help re-motivate you, and remind yourself of the names of people who could support you.

My personal reflections on Chapter 12

‹◇◇◇

You might find it helpful to write down your key personal learning points from this chapter.

* What are the key things you have learned that will help you compassionately maintain your motivation to eat well for life?

‹◇◇◇

SUMMARY

In this chapter, we have explored the process of change and, using your compassionate mind, helped you to develop an understanding of your current stage of motivation and to identify ways of supporting yourself as you move forward. We have also explored how to deal compassionately with the lapses that are inevitable as you change your eating habits, and how to treat them as important new learning opportunities, rather than see them as failures or insurmountable obstacles.

In the next chapter, we will work on the first stage of a compassionate action plan to address the practical elements of changing our eating patterns: finding out the amount and types of foods we eat, and how to provide our body with the physical activity and rest it needs to keep us healthy.

13 Working out what your body needs

In the previous chapter, we explored how to develop your motivation for working on overeating. By now I hope you are clearer about the reasons why you overeat and the intended and unintended consequences of overeating, the reasons you want to change your eating habits, and some of the blocks that may get in the way. This chapter focuses on our physical need for food, activity and rest. It will show you how to work out your own personal energy needs so that you can use this information to work out a new approach to caring for your body.

Caring about our physical wellbeing includes:

- eating as much as our body needs

- balancing our energy intake throughout the day

- providing our body with the nutrients it needs

- providing our body with foods that will help us to feel full and satisfied

- providing our body with enough physical activity to keep it healthy

- providing our body with adequate time to rest and repair itself.

Caring about our emotional needs includes:

- managing our emotional regulation systems (the 'three circles')

- developing a range of coping strategies to deal with various kinds of threat

- developing emotional resilience to manage life's challenges and setbacks

- allowing ourselves to experience joy and pleasure, including enjoying eating.

Looking after our physical needs

As we have seen, our comfort food, dieting and other eating mindsets can lead us to eat in ways that do not meet our physical needs. Unless we eat enough satisfying food on a regular basis, we are very likely to overeat (as well as to experience a whole range of physical and psychological problems), but if we regularly eat more than we need we are likely to weigh more than we need to and be at more risk of health problems. So, the ways we eat, and the amount and types of food we eat, can be critical in addressing overeating.

We are a species that evolved to be active – indeed, physical activity can have the same effect as antidepressant medication in improving our mood. But, due to the cultures we live in, many of us have become very sedentary. If we are aiming to develop a compassionate approach to our body, we also need to think about our relationship with physical activity. We need about an hour of physical activity a day that raises our heart rate but leaves us able to hold a conversation while we are doing it. However, it is important to take medical advice before you start taking more exercise, particularly if you have been inactive for a while.

Many of us lead very busy lives that do not take account of our body's needs to rest and repair. Indeed, lack of sleep has been associated with mood problems and a tendency to overeat. It's recommended that most adults have seven or eight hours' sleep a night.

Many of you reading this book will be looking to it to help them lose weight. That is absolutely OK *as long as you are actually overweight*. As we have seen, being overweight can pose physical health problems, although perhaps not as many as we are often led to believe. A compassionate approach to our body may lead us to lose weight if overeating leads us to consistently eating more than our body needs, or if we have experienced the yo-yo weight loss and gain that is usually associated with dieting. However, weight loss is not the main aim of taking a more compassionate approach to your body's needs. *The main aim is to learn to feed your body and provide it with appropriate activity to keep it as healthy as possible, and to help you to find and live with the body that your genetic history meant you to live in.* This can be a difficult journey as our emotions and eating habits can become very entangled, so it is also likely we will need to address our emotional needs along the way.

What does your body need?

Working out *exactly* what any individual's body needs is quite a complex activity. To work out your energy needs you need to take into account your:

- gender
- age

- level of activity

- weight

- height.

If you are unwell, you will also need advice from your doctor to see if this impacts your energy needs.

The higher our weight and the more activity we do, the more energy (calories) we need. For example, a forty-year-old woman who is 165 cm tall and does light activity (exercises for about an hour one to three times per week) will have calorie needs that will vary quite a bit depending on her weight. If she is 85 kg, she will need 2,125 calories per day. If she is 100 kg, she will need 2,500 calories per day. If she is 120 kg, she will need 3,000 calories per day.

The best way for you to work out your energy needs is to use an online calculator that takes age, gender, weight, height and activity levels into account. I use the online daily calorie intake calculator at bmi-calories.com. This gives suggested intake to maintain, gain or lose weight. Please remember the key aim at this stage is to maintain, not lose weight, as weight loss is likely to trigger a dieting mindset, and all the potential complications that go with it.

The number of calories we eat is only part of the story. Our body also needs a range of foods to keep us healthy. Nutritional guidelines place these foods into five categories and suggest the approximate balance between these categories that we need to help keep us healthy. These groups are:

1. starchy foods (carbohydrates)

2. fruit and vegetables

3.   meat, fish, eggs and beans (proteins)

4.   milk and dairy foods (or substitutes such as soya milk)

5.   foods containing fat and sugar.

Starchy foods include bread, cereals, potatoes, pasta, maize and cornbread; there is also starch in beans, lentils, peas, breadfruit and cassava. All these foods contain carbohydrates, which are an essential source of energy. In a healthy diet, starchy foods should make up around a third of everything we eat.

Fruit and vegetables are a vital source of vitamins and minerals, and nutritional guidelines suggest we eat five portions of them a day. One apple, banana, pear or similar-sized fruit is one portion. A slice of pineapple or melon is one portion, and three heaped tablespoons of vegetables is another. A glass of fruit juice also counts as one portion. Juice only counts as one of your five a day, though, no matter how much you drink.

Meat, fish, eggs and beans are all sources of protein, which is essential for the growth and repair of the body. Around 15 per cent of the calories we eat each day should come from protein. Meat is a good source of protein, as well as of many vitamins and minerals. Fish is another important source of protein. There is evidence that people who eat two portions or more a week of oily fish (such as sardines, mackerel, herring or salmon) are at lower risk of heart disease. That's because oily fish contain high levels of a 'good fat' called omega-3. Eggs, pulses (e.g. beans and lentils), nuts and seeds are also great sources of protein.

Milk and dairy foods (or vegetarian/vegan options), such as cheese and yoghurt, are other good sources of protein. They also contain calcium, which helps keep bones healthy.

Fats and sugar are powerful sources of energy for the body. Fat has been divided into two groups:

1. *Saturated fats* are concentrated in such foods as pies, meat products, sausages, cakes and biscuits. These can raise your cholesterol level and increase your risk of heart disease. Most of us in the West eat too much saturated fat, putting us at risk of health problems.

2. *Unsaturated fats*, on the other hand, provide us with the essential fatty acids needed to stay healthy and can actually lower your cholesterol level. Oily fish, nuts and seeds, avocados, olive oil and other vegetable oils are sources of unsaturated fat.

There are two kinds of sugar in food:

1. *Naturally occurring sugar*, in foods such as fruit and milk, tends to be released slowly from food.

2. *Added sugar* appears in processed foods such as fizzy drinks, cakes, biscuits, chocolate, pastries, ice cream and jam. It's also in some ready-made savoury foods such as pasta sauces and baked beans. This added sugar tends to be released more quickly from food and so can lead to rapid swings in blood sugar, which can leave us feeling tired and hungry.

Figure 13.1 sets out how the recommended proportions of these different types of food in a healthy diet translate into the calories you need from each type every day. These are amounts for the average, relatively inactive, woman and man; of course, if you are very physically active or heavier you will need to add additional calories to meet the increased demands on your body.

Figure 13.1 Approximate daily calorie needs and balance of food types

Food type and ideal proportion of daily calories	Calories per day for an adult female	Calories per day for an adult male
Starch (30%)	600	750
Fruit and vegetables (30%)	600	750
Protein – meat, fish, eggs and beans (15%)	300	375
Milk and dairy (15%)	300	375
Fats and sugar (10%)	200	250
Total (100%)	2,000	2,500

Figure 13.2 The Eatwell Plate

Use the Eatwell Plate to help you get the balance right.
It shows how much of what you eat should
come from each food group

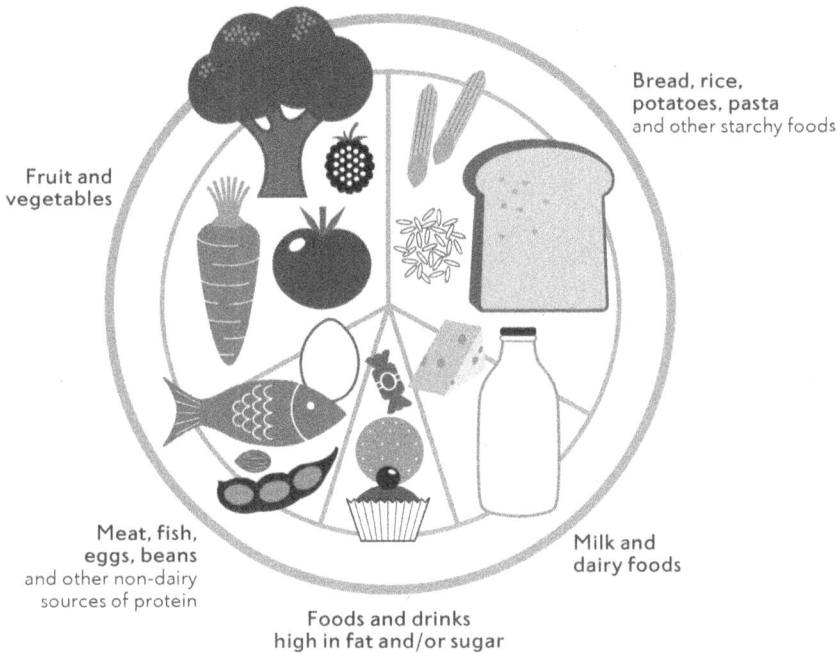

Fruit and vegetables

Bread, rice, potatoes, pasta and other starchy foods

Meat, fish, eggs, beans and other non-dairy sources of protein

Foods and drinks high in fat and/or sugar

Milk and dairy foods

Interestingly, these different food types have different effects on our satiety system. This is the system that makes us feel full and satisfied, so we know when we have eaten enough. Some foods are better than others at doing this. Protein is the most effective food for doing this, followed by starchy foods; both are better at helping us feel full and satisfied than foods whose calorie content consists largely of sugar or fat. In fact, eating sugary foods can lead to a temporary rise in blood sugar, followed by a rapid drop, leaving us hungrier, low in mood and more tired than before!

To help us overcome overeating it is really important that we eat:

- *enough* calories for our bodies' needs

- *regularly,* to avoid the blood sugar drops that provoke overeating

- a *varied* range of food, with a healthy balance between the types of food we eat.

If we do all three of these things it will help us to learn to recognise and respond to our bodies' sensations of feeling hungry and feeling full.

Moving towards balanced eating that meets your needs

Ideally, eating compassionately would mean that we understand what our body needs and when it needs it, and allow ourselves to enjoy the foods we like in a way that does not affect our health or lead to overeating. That can feel like a really tall order if we have been struggling with overeating, or denying ourselves food, for any length of time. Sometimes even thinking about this as a goal can lead us to give up, believing that this *may* be possible for some people but certainly isn't for us!

Well, if you're thinking this, you certainly won't be alone. Remember, our see-food-and-eat-it brain, and the comfort eating, dieting and other eating mindsets we develop, may take us a long way from compassionate eating. So, although this may be our goal, it is unlikely that any of us will be able to do this 100 per cent of the time. The good news is that occasionally eating in a less compassionate way (for example, overindulging in the holidays) is something that our body can cope with relatively well; it just can't cope if we do it a lot of the time.

Many people I have worked with have found it very helpful to have a structure to guide them in learning to eat compassionately. This involves putting some time into planning what and when we are going to eat, and then gradually learning to recognise our body's signals for hunger and fullness, and to respond to these. Making these changes can trigger a whole range of thoughts and feelings that can stop us from compassionately caring for our bodies. We will explore ways to work on these in more detail in the next chapter.

Working out what you're eating now

In the early stages of learning to eat compassionately you will need to devote a little time to working out what you are currently eating, and how this compares to what you need. This can be a little unnerving at first, especially if you have been used to calorie counting as part of a dieting mindset or if you are not used to being aware of what you eat. However, if you are going to work out what your body needs, you will need to know how much energy you take in, how much energy you use up, and how the types of food you eat relate to the types of food your body needs.

If you have worked through the book to this point, you will already have had a go at keeping an eating diary. We can now use this, along with a calorie-counting book, website or app, to estimate your energy needs and your energy intake. There are many commercial and open-access resources that give the calorie values of a wide range of foods. Many also tell you how many calories you use up doing different kinds of activity/exercise. I suggest that you look at a few so you can choose one that you find easy to use.

Like all tools, knowledge about the calories in the food we eat and the energy we use can potentially have some unintended consequences. These include:

- activating our dieting mindset

- reminding us of negative experiences in the past with calorie counting

- becoming obsessed with the calories we eat

- using calorie estimating to beat ourselves up for being greedy, out of control, etc.

It is really important that you explore and manage these possibilities from the perspective of your compassionate mind. Take a little time to engage your soothing system; then, when you are ready, bring your compassionate mind online. Allow yourself to experience its care and warmth for you, and then gently try to 'step into' its shoes. Imagine that you truly want to offer yourself the benefits of its strength, courage and wisdom in exploring the next two exercises.

Exercise 13.1: Identifying difficulties in calorie estimating

Allow your compassionate mind to identify any difficulties it can foresee if you were to work out the calories you have eaten, then jot them down in the space provided:

Exercise 13.2: My compassionate thoughts and actions for managing estimating my energy intake

Once you are aware of these risks, you can then use your compassionate mind to help you to develop a plan to manage them. Please remember that the aim of recording calories is to help you to understand and to care for your body's needs; it is not about losing weight or beating yourself up for overeating. If you notice your critical mindset chipping in, it is really important to slow down and return to your compassionate mind before you go on. You may wish to do this in the form of a compassionate letter, or just jot the main points in the space provided:

Spending a short period of your life becoming more aware of what you eat, and learning to eat in a way that cares for your body's needs, can be really worth the time and effort. People I have worked with have told me that this knowledge gives them control over what and how they want to eat and makes it far easier to manage the biological urges that used to cause them to overeat. The good news is that you will only need to estimate your calories in detail once during the whole programme, when you are working out your first meal plan. You can use the information you have gathered from your diaries so far to do this. Ideally, use at least two weeks' worth of food diary records, particularly if there are big variations in how much you eat or how much activity you do.

It is a lot easier to estimate your energy balance when you have a meal plan in place, as you can simply add or subtract calorie estimates for food you eat in addition to the plan or for foods you leave out, as well as increases or decreases in your activity levels.

You can use the following guidelines to help you with this task:

- Estimate calories. You don't need to weigh out to the gram everything that you eat – a good estimate is usually enough.

- Make a note of all the physical activities you do in fifteen-minute episodes.

- Make a note of the types of food you eat, and approximately how many calories per day of each of the five main food types you eat (see page 340–1).

Let's think about what this would look like in practice by exploring Alison's diary again. Take a look back at Figure 9.2 (page 264).

We will presume that Alison is forty years old, 171 cm tall (5 foot 6 inches) and weighs 73 kg (11 stone 8lb). She was not particularly active on this Monday (23 March), so her energy requirement would have been around 2,090 calories. However, if Alison were more active, as she was on the Tuesday, we would have to raise her energy need to take this into account. For example, on Tuesday she spent four hours doing housework, and two hours doing exercise. She can use a calorie-counting book, website or app to work out her energy needs for three hours of housework (720 calories) and two hours doing exercise (two aerobic classes at the gym = 840 calories). We will not include one hour of the housework, as this would have been included in Alison's routine energy needs. So, on Tuesday, Alison needed around 3,650 calories to meet her energy needs.

You can see from this that physical activity can make a big difference to how much we need to eat. It is really important to take this into account when we are trying to understand daily fluctuations in our energy needs, and how hungry we are likely to be.

If we go back to Alison's eating diary for Monday 23 March, we can add up approximately how many calories she ate and drank:

- 1 bowl of cereal with skimmed milk and sugar = 200 calories

- 2 slices of toast and butter = 300 calories

- 15 ginger biscuits = 750 calories

- Burger meal (small cheeseburger, no chips), large milkshake = 700 calories

- 4 (small) glasses of red wine = 350 calories

- Takeaway meal (pizza, 4 slices) = 1,280 calories

- Individual tub of ice cream = 180 calories

- 3 cups of tea with skimmed milk = 30 calories

Total calories = 3,790

This would have been only a little more than she needed on Tuesday but was 1,700 calories more than the 2,090 her body needed on Monday. One of the typical patterns that we can fall into when we overeat is to try to make up for it the next day (hence Alison's very active day on Tuesday after she had overeaten on Monday). Although Alison's energy intake across the two days more or less balances out, the problem was that she swung between overeating one day and then not eating enough for her needs the next day. By the time she reached Wednesday she was back to overeating because she became very hungry after leaving herself so short of the energy she needed on Tuesday. We will explore how to address this issue when we come to meal planning in the next chapter.

The other interesting thing that Alison discovered from her diary was that most of her calories came from foods high in fat and sugar, such as biscuits, or high in carbohydrate, like cereal, bread and pizza. She also tended to have quite a lot of dairy products, such as milk and milkshakes, and a significant percentage of her calories came from alcohol. Her protein intake was relatively small (mainly the meat in her burger), and she had no fruit or vegetables on Monday. The difficulty here was that the high-energy foods she ate were also the foods that she found least filling, and so she tended to eat more of them.

Ideally, Alison needed to significantly increase her intake of foods that were less high in energy but would help fill her up (such as fruit and vegetables). She also needed to swap her high-energy foods for others that included more protein, which again would be more filling than fatty and sugary foods such as biscuits. With time and perseverance Alison was able to make significant changes in her energy intake and to change the balance of the food types she ate. She also learned to develop other ways to cope with the low moods and distress that she had got used to relieving by eating. Alison learned to lower her 'emotional temperature' by introducing a number of self-soothing activities into her daily routine – such as ensuring she had a 'me time' bath every evening. She also practised using her safe place imagery to help her regain some emotional stability when she got upset. In fact, she became so good at this she was able to be soothed by just imagining a peaceful beach for a couple of seconds. Alison also built a number of distractions into her routine, even including her partner in salsa dance classes.

As she grew in confidence in her ability to soothe and distract herself from some of the painful feelings that triggered her over-eating, Alison decided to tolerate these feelings long enough to resist the urge to overeat. This gave her time to change her eating while she explored what she was upset about. She was able to use her compassionate formulation to make sense of a number of painful events in her past, as well as her dissatisfaction with her job. She allowed herself to grieve her previous difficult experiences but decided to move on with her life, letting go of some difficult relationships and changing her career to one she found more fulfilling. Of course, she still overate occasionally, but she was able to acknowledge these instances as part of the normal eating experience and no longer beat herself up or turn it into a cycle of comfort eating and dieting. Her weight gradually stabilised, and she learned to appreciate her body and enjoy eating.

Like many of us, Alison tended to estimate the calories she had eaten in relation to how she felt about food. For example, she believed her biscuits, which were high in fat and sugar, contained far fewer calories than her breakfast, as breakfast tended to be more filling. She was feeling quite upset when she had her burger, and greedy when she had her takeaway, so she tended to overestimate what she had eaten on these occasions. She often associated feeling full with feeling greedy or having overeaten. She found it really helpful to work out realistic calorie estimates for these eating episodes and to see how they differed from her 'feeling based' calorie estimates.

Working out your energy balance

Our energy balance is the difference between the amount of energy we take in and the amount we need to fuel our bodily systems and whatever else we do. Most people who overeat will have a positive energy balance (they eat more than they need), but on some days they may have a negative energy balance (eating less than they need). A long-term positive balance leads to weight gain, while severe short- and medium-term negative balances tend to lead to overeating. In this section we are interested in helping you develop a more neutral energy balance, to help reduce overeating that is based on feeling hungry. This will also help to stabilise your weight so that you do not need to get into a dieting mindset to manage it.

As we have already seen, there are two elements to our daily energy needs: our basic needs and the energy we use up above our normal needs (for example, through doing housework, walking, or formal exercise such as playing football or going to the gym).

It's best to work out our energy balance over a week, as it can fluctuate quite a lot from one day to the next. The easiest way to do this is to calculate intake and energy used for each day and then add them up at the end of the week. You can record these details in Worksheets 13 and 14 overleaf. The first of these can help you keep a daily record of your energy balance, while the second helps you keep a weekly summary. Please read the remaining text in this chapter before you begin to fill in either of the worksheets.

Worksheet 13: Food intake and energy balance daily record

Food eaten	Approximate energy intake (calories)	Main food type (e.g. starch, fruit/ veg, protein, dairy, sugar/ fat)	Activity log and approx- imate energy used

Worksheet 14: Food intake and energy balance summary

	Mon.	Tues.	Wed.	Thurs.	Fri.	Sat.	Sun.	Weekly summary
Total calorie intake								
Starch								
Fruit and vegetables								
Protein								
Dairy								
Sugar and fat								
Alcohol								
Base energy need + extra for energy expended in activity								
Energy balance (= calorie intake – energy need)								

As well as the amount of food we eat, we are interested in eating more of the foods that can keep us healthy and feeling satisfied. So, the worksheets also give you space to record what you are eating and the food type it belongs to. You can then work out the approximate proportion of each type of food you eat in your total intake each day and have a weekly summary (as it can be difficult to eat enough of each food group every day).

We are also interested in the amount of activity we undertake, as the other half of our energy balance equation is how much energy we use up. We can then work out whether we are eating more or less than we need each day, and across the week.

When you have all this information you will be able to use it as the basis for the next stage in changing your eating habits, which is planning your meals to incorporate changes in the amounts and types of foods you eat. This will be the focus of the next chapter.

You can see an example of how to fill in a weekly summary sheet in Figure 13.3 opposite. This is based on Alison's diary for Monday 23 March.

Exercise 13.3 will take you through some steps to help you complete Worksheet 14.

The blank worksheets have spaces for you to record the food you eat, your approximate energy intake (in calories) from it, the type of food it belongs to, and any physical activity. This includes formal exercise, but also day-to-day things like housework or walking. You can note down your calorie totals (both consumed and used) to arrive at energy balance figures for each day, and then for the whole week.

Figure 13.3 Alison's food intake and energy balance summary, Monday 23 March

	Mon.	Tues.	Wed.	Thurs.	Fri.	Sat.	Sun.	Weekly summary
Total calorie intake	3,790							
Starch	1,920							
Fruit and vegetables	0							
Protein	100							
Dairy	640							
Sugar and fat	780							
Alcohol	350							
Base energy need + extra for energy expended in activity	2,090 No extra							
Energy balance (= calorie intake – energy need)	+1,700							

We are particularly interested here not only in whether you end up with a positive or negative energy balance but also in what food types you're mostly eating. You can use the Eatwell Plate and the information in Figure 13.2 to guide you in allocating food types. For example, ginger biscuits do contain a lot of starch, but they are included in the 'Sugar and fat' column for Alison's worksheet because this is where biscuits appear on the Eatwell Plate.

When you are working out your energy balance you will need to spend a little time reflecting on the types of activity you did each day. Many people are surprised by just how active they are, and in itself this can sometimes account for some apparent 'overeating'. As we saw in Chapter 2, if you are lying in bed doing nothing all day, you will need around 1,600 calories just to 'tick over' without doing any activity at all. You can use the daily calorie intake calculator at bmi-calories.com to calculate your overall needs based on your activity levels. If you are more active than this, you will need to increase your energy intake accordingly – keeping roughly to the same proportions of food types as set out in the Eatwell Plate. For example, if you do an extra hour in the gym you may need an extra 300 calories, ideally in the form of 90 calories of starch, 90 calories of fruit and vegetables, 45 calories of meat, fish eggs, or beans, 45 calories of dairy products and 30 calories of fat and sugar during the course of the day. You will also need some extra fluid to replace what you will lose though perspiration – and a bit of rest to let your body recover!

When you are familiar with Worksheet 14 and have looked though Alison's example in Figure 13.3 you are ready to think about doing Exercise 13.3.

The key to this is to use your compassionate mind to explore your food diary and complete your worksheet with an approach of gentle curiosity.

- *Gentleness* is important because this exercise can lead to us feeling disappointed, angry or ashamed of what and how we eat, so we really do need to be kind to ourselves and compassionate with the struggles we have with eating. Your compassionate mind can use your personal compassionate formulation to help you understand why you eat the way you do, and to support and value your commitment to changing the way you eat.

- *Curiosity* is also important, because exploring the types and amounts of food we eat can often provide us with new insights into the areas we feel we can begin to work on. Many people have found that taking a kindly enquiring perspective can help them overcome their usual pattern of either avoiding thinking about what they eat or attacking themselves for what and how they eat.

Remember, you only need to work out your energy balance and the types of food you have eaten in detail once – to give you an idea of your pattern to help you to work out your first meal plan. Doing it in this degree of detail for any longer will become a chore at the very least, and at worst can be counterproductive, as constantly counting the calories of everything you eat is likely to activate your dieting mindset. Once you've done this one-off exercise, it is far more helpful to begin to plan your eating in advance, and then review it at the end of the week, making a note of any times when you have varied from your plan, to help you refine it or to address things that have led to overeating, as part of the plan for the following week.

Only begin Exercise 13.3 when you feel emotionally ready and practically prepared to start to make changes. The exercise can take about two hours in total, so you need to set aside time when you can work on it either all in one go or in several shorter sessions. It can also activate difficult thoughts and feelings and memories in us, particularly if we have dieted a lot in the past or are critical of our eating. So, we will need our compassionate mind to guide us, support us through the process and help us to tolerate any distress that the activity may cause us. Your compassionate mind will be wise enough to know how much of this you can manage at any one time. It can also be helpful to have some self-soothing or other distress management activities pre-arranged for when you finish the exercise.

Exercise 13.3: Working out your own energy balance

Begin by using your safe place image or soothing breathing rhythm to bring your soothing system into play. It is common for people doing this exercise to find that their mind wanders even more frequently than usual; this may be because you have associated looking at what you eat with the urge to diet or self-criticise. Remember to use the motto 'notice and return' to gently refocus your attention on the task in hand.

When you can feel that your soothing system is online, you are ready to move on to the next stage – activating your compassionate mind. Allow yourself to experience its compassion for your courage and wisdom in taking on the task of exploring your diary. What sort of things would it say to support you? How would it encourage you to explore it compassionately rather than using it as a way of motivating you to eat less, or punishing you for eating too much?

You can then explore your eating diary from the perspective of your compassionate mind. Some people find this very challenging and prefer to imagine their compassionate companion exploring the diary, but imagining it belongs to someone else they care about, therefore reading in a more detached way, but still with gentle, compassionate curiosity. You may find it easier just to work through one day at a time, and to do the exercise over several days, before you add up your week and summarise the information on the worksheet.

However you do this, take your time over it. It is an important part of the groundwork for all the other things you will do to change your relationship with food, eating and your body, so you deserve to spend some time doing it at a pace you can manage.

When you have finished filling in Worksheet 14, you can explore what your compassionate mind would say about what you have learned, and what changes you could work on with regard to the amount you eat, the types of food you eat and your activity levels. You may wish to jot these thoughts down, perhaps in the form of a compassionate letter, to guide the efforts to address your overeating.

My personal reflections on Chapter 13

You might find it helpful to write down your key personal learning points from this chapter.

- What were your first thoughts when reviewing your eating and activity?

- What ways have you found to help you estimate the energy you need?

- What types of food do you need to eat more of/less of?

SUMMARY

This chapter has explored what being compassionate with our bodies' needs means, particularly in terms of energy, activity and rest. We have explored a way of using two weeks' worth of records from your food diary to help you work out your energy balance and the types of food you eat. You can now use this as the basis for developing your plan for changing your eating and of course working on the thoughts and feelings that lead to over-eating, or that may follow from changing your eating. The next two chapters will guide you through a step-by-step approach to doing this compassionately.

14 Developing a new way of eating – a practical guide

This chapter brings together all the work you have done so far, to create a practical plan for addressing overeating and caring for your body. It shows you how to establish a basic structure for eating that includes managing foods that can put you at risk of overeating. As always, the key is to use your compassionate mind, based on wisdom and a genuine desire to be encouraging and supportive, to guide you.

The six-step programme: an outline

In the early stages of building a new relationship with food and your body, you will need to spend time planning when, how and what you are going to eat. The longer you spend doing this – three to six months is probably a good period to aim for – the more likely you are to establish a new eating routine. Then, gradually, you can become less strict with your meal plans, experiment with a wider range of foods, and learn to respond to your experiences of being hungry and full.

Many people confuse meal planning with dieting. Meal planning is not a diet. It is about making changes in our eating pattern, and later in the amounts and types of food we eat. It does this by taking away the option of eating less later if (for any reason) we overeat, as we know we will still stick to eating the next meal we have planned. It can also help us to change some of the common features of chaotic eating patterns, such as leaving long periods between meals or eating very frequently, that can put us out of touch with our feelings of hunger and fullness.

Our new way of eating involves learning to be more mindful of the influences that can lead to overeating. It is broken down into six steps:

1. Establishing a regular eating pattern.

2. Reducing our intake of high-risk foods that trigger overeating.

3. Balancing our energy intake with our energy needs.

4. Developing a healthy nutritional balance.

5. Learning to respond to our hunger and fullness.

6. Learning to enjoy food and eating.

Each step will help you learn more about your relationship with overeating. It is best to start with step 1 and work through all the steps at a pace you feel comfortable with. As with any new skill, you should only move on when you feel relatively confident that you can manage each step. A good rule of thumb is to move up a step when you can manage it for about five days in a week, and to move back a step if you are struggling for two or three days in a row.

This chapter will take you through the first two steps of the programme; the next chapter will cover the remaining four.

Step 1: Establishing a regular eating pattern

We will start with establishing a pattern of eating regularly as the basis for all the other changes we will introduce. Regular eating patterns tend to reduce the body's urge to overeat and help to balance out high and low levels of blood sugar, which have a powerful influence on our appetite and moods.

If you're going to eat regularly, this means planning when to eat rather than eating when you feel like it! And yes, there will be rules for you to follow. If you have struggled with overeating for some time, you'll probably need to stick to these for a while. They are:

1. Plan when you are going to eat.

2. Eat by the clock, not your feelings.

3. Eat every three to four hours.

4. Do not skip an eating episode.

5. Do not add an eating episode.

These rules may look a bit daunting at first, even a little authoritarian, and perhaps impossible to stick to. But, don't worry, although it may take a little time to establish them, most people do manage over time. Of course, you may need to bend the rules occasionally – but the more quickly you can establish a regular eating pattern, with spaced out eating episodes, the easier it will be to stop overeating. At this point, you are not aiming to change the amounts or types of food that you eat.

To set out your eating plan and record how you keep to it, you will need to use the eating diary that we first saw in Chapter 9. As we discussed earlier, reviewing our diaries can unintentionally lead us into a dieting or self-critical mindset. So please be aware of these potential obstacles and prepare yourself to overcome them by ensuring that you plan your eating and review your diary with your compassionate mind. You can begin by engaging your soothing system; then, when you are ready, bring your compassionate mind online. Focus on your feelings of wisdom and encouragement throughout this next exercise, which will take you through reviewing your eating diary to drawing up a regular eating plan.

Exercise 14.1: Planning to eat more regularly

Start by picking a 'typical day' from your diary – not one of your worst days for overeating, nor one when you are dieting. What do you notice about the times that you eat? Are there gaps between them of more than three to four hours? Or do you find it difficult to leave gaps – for example, do you eat every couple of hours, or even find yourself grazing all day? If you notice either of these trends, try to use your compassionate mind to explore the key questions in Worksheet 15. You can use your compassionate eating formulation and your analysis of overeating and the three emotion regulation systems from Chapter 11 to help you. You might want to use your compassionate mind to review these questions at the end of each day for the first few weeks, to explore why meal planning may be difficult for you.

Worksheet 15: Making sense of my struggles with meal planning

Why don't I space the meals I eat?	
How does it help me to eat more (or less) frequently than my body needs?	
Would I encourage other people in my life that I care about to space their eating the way I do?	
How could I encourage myself to eat more regularly? What could I do or say to help me do this?	

When you feel ready, try to develop a daily eating plan based upon the amount and types of food you currently eat. The aim is to break this down into between five and seven eating episodes during the day. Try to eat every three and a half to four hours, starting with breakfast within about thirty minutes of getting up, and ending with a light snack just before you go to bed.

Draw on the wisdom of your compassionate mind to help you set realistic and achievable expectations about when you are going to eat. It will understand that you may still feel the need to over-eat and will not expect you to give this up until you are ready. So, at this stage, if you still need to overeat – for example, to help you manage a difficult feeling – that's OK. However, try to do this in a more planned way. For example, you may really want a big tub of ice cream as a comfort food, but instead of coming home and raiding the freezer an hour before you have planned to eat, try to delay your urge and have your ice cream at a time when you have scheduled a meal and when your body is likely to be hungry. In Worksheet 16 I have provided a seven-episode eating plan for you to fill in, followed by a completed example from Alison.

Worksheet 16: Regular eating

Meal or snack	Time and place, and who with	Food and drink to be taken	Comments (Including any problems in keeping to my plan, any solutions for these problems or changes to the plan)
Breakfast			
Mid–morning snack			
Lunch			

Mid-afternoon snack			
Evening meal			
Evening snack			
Supper			

Figure 14.1 Alison's regular eating worksheet

Meal or snack	Time and place, and who with	Food and drink to be taken	Comments (Including any problems in keeping to my plan, any solutions for these problems or changes to the plan)
Breakfast	Get up at 7 a.m. Eat at 7.30 a.m. With partner	Cereal and milk 2 slices of toast Cup of tea, milk, 1 sugar	
Mid–morning snack	10.30 a.m. At my desk at work, talking to colleague	Cup of tea, milk, 1 sugar 5 ginger biscuits	
Lunch	1 p.m. At burger bar with colleague	Burger meal and shake	

Mid-afternoon snack	4.30 p.m. At work, in staff room with other staff	Cup of tea, milk, 1 sugar 5 ginger biscuits		
Evening meal	7.15 p.m. At home, with partner, at the dinner table	Takeaway (pizza) Individual tub of ice cream 2 glasses of red wine		
Evening snack	10.30 p.m. At home with partner, living room watching TV	5 ginger biscuits 2 glasses of red wine		
Supper	No supper as going to bed early			

Regular eating, even on its own, can have a positive impact on overeating for some people, so as you start working on this you may want to look back over your diary each week to see if your eating has improved.

In Figure 14.1 you can see a completed example of Worksheet 16 for Alison. It's an early worksheet, before she made significant changes to the amount and type of foods she ate.

When you look at Alison's worksheet clearly, drinking four glasses of wine every night wouldn't be very healthy; however, Alison only drank on one evening a week, and this was the one night when she spent time with her partner watching a film. Alison acknowledged that she would rather drink less, and over time she managed to space it a little more across the week, while keeping well within recommended limits. However, in the early stages of learning to eat regularly she did not think she could do this and change her 'drinking for fun and relaxation' mindset at the same time. This is not uncommon, and it is always important to use your compassionate mind to guide how far you can go with making changes at any one time.

You may also notice that Alison planned both when and where she ate. She had noticed that eating alone placed her at greater risk of overeating and also left her quite vulnerable to the waves of emotion that often accompanied eating. She found that planning to eat in the company of others helped to provide her with some emotional support (even though the people she ate with at work were unaware that they did this) and also helped to distract her from the very self-critical thoughts she had when she was eating.

Interestingly, Alison found that this level of planning took away a lot of her anxiety about eating and gave her a greater sense of control over her appetite. It also helped her to recognise how different mindsets during the day influenced her and how the people she was with could also affect her urges to eat.

Some people find it difficult to establish a regular eating plan. This is not surprising given the obstacles that can arise from having to rearrange when and how we eat, let alone the emotional reasons for eating in the way we have got used to doing. The next exercise is designed to help you explore any blocks you may have, and to develop a plan and alternative compassionate thoughts to help you address those blocks.

Exercise 14.2: Managing blocks to eating regularly

The first step is to imagine that you are going to start eating regularly from tomorrow. This can be quite exciting; however, you might have a lot of 'yes, buts' or imagine the problems that might arise when you start. These problems could be practical (e.g. 'I don't have food in the house') or related to your thoughts and feelings (e.g. 'I am worried that if I can't comfort eat, I won't be able to cope'). Write these down in the left-hand column of Worksheet 17.

Worksheet 17: Managing blocks to regular eating

Practical and emotional blocks to managing regular eating	Compassionate things I can say to myself or do to get past the block

Take a little time to feel compassion for yourself, either from 'you at your best' or from your compassionate companion. Then allow yourself to feel compassion for the blocks that you may encounter. Remember, it is not your fault that these arise: maybe there are very real obstacles in the way, or maybe thinking of making these changes has activated your threat system in some way and this is your brain's way of trying to protect you from potential harms. Take a little time to explore why these blocks may have arisen and perhaps try to write the reasons down underneath the blocks themselves on the worksheet.

Finally, imagine how you would feel if you could work through these blocks and manage the feelings that might arise as you did so. You may then wish to add in the right-hand column anything that you could do or say to yourself to help you overcome these blocks and begin to eat regularly. There is a completed example of the worksheet to help you in Figure 14.2.

When you begin to space your meals out more regularly, you may find that this too can be difficult at times, or that it may provoke painful thoughts and feelings. Keep a note of these in your eating diary, because when you review it these notes will help you understand what works in favour of your eating more regularly and what tends to obstruct you.

Remember: you are likely to have setbacks along the way. Each new block you encounter is a sign, not of failure but of your courage in making changes, and an opportunity for you to learn more about how your eating works.

Figure 14.2 Managing blocks to regular eating – an example

Practical and emotional blocks to managing regular eating	Compassionate things I can say to myself or do to get past the block
I get so peckish – especially if I see food on TV.	*This very understandable. I do tend to get peckish a lot in the evening, sometimes because I have not eaten as often as my body needs. Eating more regularly might make this a bit easier. TV is designed to make us peckish, after all – otherwise why make adverts?! However, before reaching for that unplanned snack, I can take a breath, bring on my compassionate mind and consider how I would feel if I resisted.*
I am so busy I don't really stop for lunch – well, few people in the office do.	*This is hard – especially when other people at work don't stop. However, I do deserve the time to eat, and I will try to reschedule my work so that I can. Perhaps I could even encourage a few other people to join me.*

Step 2: Compassionately reducing trigger foods to overeating

The next step is to reduce your risk of being tempted to overeat out of habit or as a way of managing your feelings. The compassionate element here is to work out what you can actually manage without triggering your dieting mind, being overwhelmed by feelings or depriving yourself of these foods as a way of punishing yourself. This step can be trickier than it looks, but it has the advantage of not requiring you to count calories or plan your meals.

First, identify the types of foods that are most likely to put you at risk of overeating. These may be foods that you associate with comfort eating, or foods that you really enjoy but find it hard to stop eating once you've started.

Returning to Alison's worksheet (Figure 14.1), we can see that she had several foods that were associated with emotional comfort (e.g. ginger biscuits) and some foods that she really enjoyed (e.g. burgers or pizza). Some of these fell into both categories, in that she enjoyed them and also ate them to 'treat' herself for having been upset. Sometimes Alison would eat sweets when she felt angry with herself. This didn't really give her comfort, and she didn't really enjoy them either. After a while she realised that she ate these when she felt very self-critical because she knew they were 'bad' for her, and she felt she didn't deserve to eat more healthily or to be happy – in other words, they became ways of punishing herself. Of course, this was something she really needed to work on, and she gradually managed to stop doing this as she became less self-critical and more self-compassionate.

You can use your own eating diary to work out the types of food that put you at risk of overeating. You can then list them in Worksheet 18, putting them into one or more of the four categories according to why you tend to eat too much of them. Figure 14.3 gives you an example of how to do this using Alison's observations.

Worksheet 18: My high-risk foods for overeating

Food	Comfort food? Yes/No	Enjoyable food? Yes/No	Treat food? Yes/No	Self-punishing food? Yes/No

Figure 14.3 Alison's high-risk foods for overeating

Food	Comfort food? Yes/No	Enjoyable food? Yes/No	Treat food? Yes/No	Self-punishing food? Yes/No
Ginger biscuits	Yes	Not really	No	No
Burger	No	Yes	Yes	No
Pizza	No	Yes	Yes	No
Sweets	No	Yes	No	No
Wine	No	Yes	Yes	No

Next, you can begin to work on reducing the amounts of these foods that you eat. Try doing this in four stages, as outlined below.

1. Don't tell yourself you are not allowed to have them!

This is really important. Humans have a tendency to want what they can't have the minute they are told they can't have it! Remember when I asked you to imagine I'd said you couldn't go to the toilet until you'd finished reading the chapter? This urge to do whatever we're told we can't do becomes even stronger if we feel we are denying ourselves something really important to us, such as something we enjoy, or something that gives us comfort, or even something that punishes us. Again, the more compassionate we are to ourselves about these urges, the easier it is to manage them.

2. Work out what the minimum amount of this type of food is that you can eat.

The key here is not to stop eating this food entirely. You may still have the need to comfort eat for some time and will still want to eat many foods because you enjoy them. As you work on changing your eating habits and learn new ways to deal with your feelings, you will also be gradually working on changing the emotional meaning of foods – particularly foods you habitually use to comfort or punish yourself. However, at this stage we are trying to help you reduce the amount of these that you eat, while, at the same time, you learn to tolerate your feelings.

To begin with, work out how much of the food you need to eat to get the emotional response that you want. Aim to have only this much of the food available to you at any one time. Of course, you may be tempted to buy more when it has gone. However, this approach will at least mean that you have time to stop and think before you do, so that you can understand your urges and give yourself some time to work with them.

3. Gradually reduce the amount of this type of food and learn to tolerate your emotions.

The aim here is to allow yourself enough of the food to take the edge off your emotions, and to learn to tolerate them a little more. To see how this works in practice, let's go back to Alison. Alison found that ten biscuits tended to be enough for her to feel comforted, and after this she did not feel any more comfort from the biscuits, even if she ate another twenty. So initially she decided to keep ten comfort biscuits that she could use if she needed them. She could only have ten, so that meant that the rest of the packet got thrown away. It was a waste of money, but she would have wasted her money on extra biscuits anyway as they did not provide her with extra comfort, and overeating by eating them all did not stop her eating again later.

After several weeks of doing this, Alison felt that she could gradually reduce her reliance on biscuits for emotional comfort. So, she decided to reduce the total by one biscuit at a time. Alison managed to do this, and although she felt some distress when she did not have as many biscuits as usual, she felt she could cope as long as she had her safety net of a smaller number of biscuits.

The extent and rate at which you reduce your comfort eating and switch to a healthier balance of foods will be personal to you. It is also important to bear in mind that even when we are eating in a more balanced way we are still allowed to eat and enjoy foods that we have used as comfort foods in the past; the key is just to change our relationship with them, so we are not using them to manage our emotional life. We'll be looking more at this in the next chapter.

4. Increase the delay between the urge to eat your specific food and eating it.

This is similar to reducing your intake slowly, in that you are learning to sit with your feelings for a time, and finding other ways to manage them. You may recall that we explored mindfulness in Chapter 5. This is a good time to become more mindful by learning to notice what your feelings are – not to change them, necessarily, but to notice them.

You might also find it useful to write your feelings down. What is going on for you when you turn away from comfort eating or say 'no' to those foods you love? Rather than eating your feelings away you will have written compassionately about them, helping you to understand them better, and becoming kinder and gentler with them. You may also find that writing about them lowers the power of the eating urges.

Alison did not feel she could give up biscuits as a comfort food entirely, so when she got down to seven biscuits she worked instead on delaying when she would eat them. Initially she decided that she could only manage one minute of feeling distressed before she ate her biscuits. Gradually she built this up to five minutes, which gave her time to put other coping strategies in place.

The key issue here is learning to become mindful of what we eat and why we eat it. Minimising the amount of these foods and delaying when you eat them can help you be more in control of the quantity you eat, but more importantly gives you time to reflect on your reasons for overeating.

If you eat to treat yourself or because you enjoy a particular type of food, by all means let yourself have these feelings. But take time over the taste, texture and smell of the food rather than gobbling it down. Eat it in a way that is within your control and only eat the amount you need to eat to have these feelings.

You may have heard someone refer to some foods as their 'guilty pleasure'. If you feel like this about, say, chocolate, you could work on reducing the feelings of guilt so that chocolate becomes something you can eat and enjoy. You may well find that you get more satisfaction and enjoyment from one chocolate that you eat slowly, focusing on savouring the taste and texture, than you get from eating a whole box while watching TV! What's happening here is that the feeling of being a naughty child has changed to that of being an adult, in control, who is allowed to feel pleasure.

My personal reflections on Chapter 14

You might find it helpful to write down your key personal learning points from this chapter.

- What were your first thoughts about developing a meal plan?

- What do you think your main blocks to meal planning will be, and what can you do or say to yourself to help manage them compassionately?

SUMMARY

This chapter has explored the first practical steps that you can take towards changing your eating habits. We have explored how you can begin to eat more regularly, and ways to think about and address some of the potential obstacles to this. We have also explored how you can allow yourself to slowly reduce the types and amount of food that can trigger your overeating. These first steps can help you to manage some of the biological highs and lows that come with chaotic eating patterns, and to tolerate and understand your urges to overeat.

The key here is to be compassionate with your attempts to eat more regularly and your urges to overeat. When you feel that you can manage a regular eating pattern and have a little more control over and understanding of the foods that can trigger overeating, you are ready to move towards the second phase: changing the amounts and types of food that you eat and learning to respond to your body's needs. We will look at these steps in the next chapter.

15 Towards a new way of eating – the final steps

In Chapter 14, we worked through the first two steps of a programme to establish new eating habits by spacing your eating and reducing your intake of foods that are likely to lead to overeating. In this chapter, we will move on to cover the remaining four steps: planning what you eat to meet your energy needs; improving the nutritional balance of what you eat; learning to respond to your body's signals for hunger and fullness; and, finally, learning to enjoy eating and caring for your body's needs.

The benefits of meal planning

Meal planning can be tricky to begin with, and I am often asked whether the effort is worth it. It does take some time, certainly, but, in my experience, it is crucial to resolving overeating. Most people who don't overeat tend to eat regularly and have a good idea of the types and amount of food they will eat and when. If you don't have a 'sense' of this – and many people who overeat don't – then it's certainly worth learning to acquire it, which is what meal planning is all about.

It is important to recognise that meal planning is not an end in itself. None of us want to have to plan exactly what we are going to eat and when we will eat it for the rest of our lives! Meal planning is the basis for helping you separate emotional overeating (because you're angry, for example) from biologically driven overeating (because you're hungry). It can also:

- give us a clear idea of what we intend to eat
- provide a structure to eating
- help avoid chaotic eating patterns
- match our energy intake to our energy needs so we are less likely to be hungry
- give us a baseline from which to make changes in the types and amount of food we eat
- help us take into account changes in our daily energy needs
- help us identify and work with times when we eat 'off plan'
- retrain our body to experience feeling hungry and feeling full.

You are likely to need to plan your eating for between three and six months. Gradually you will develop a menu of foods that you can eat regularly that will meet your nutritional needs and won't lead to overeating – this will make planning (and shopping!) a lot easier – and can then move towards eating in response to the signals your body gives you, rather than according to your plan. Please remember that it should be based around foods that you enjoy, help you feel full and keep you healthy.

Potential problems with meal planning

Many people encounter problems in developing a meal plan and putting it into practice. These may include:

- not knowing how much of a particular food to eat
- feeling too constrained by the plan

- difficulty keeping to the plan when other people are around

- difficulty keeping to the plan when on holiday or visiting others.

It's useful to identify any problems you think might crop up and have some ideas about how to deal with them before you actually start on your plan. The next exercise will help you to do this.

Exercise 15.1: Identifying potential problems with meal planning

Please consider any problems you think you might face and write them down in the space provided. I have given you space for four problems; these might be psychological (e.g. 'I feel too controlled by a plan') or practical. There are likely to be more than this as you try to put your meal plan into practice. That is perfectly normal, and part of the work is identifying these problems and working through them as they arise. For now, just focus on anything that you can think of that might make it difficult to follow your plan on day one.

- _____

- _____

- _____

- _____

You can now write these in the left-hand column of Worksheet 19. Then, using your compassionate mind to guide you, as you did when you started to plan to eat regularly, think about what you might do or say to yourself to overcome these problems, and write your suggestions in the right-hand column. Figure 15.1 shows an example of a completed worksheet that may help you.

Worksheet 19: Dealing with blocks to meal planning

Practical and emotional blocks to managing a meal plan	Compassionate things I can say to myself or do to help me manage my meal plan

Figure 15.1 Dealing with blocks to meal planning – an example

Practical and emotional blocks to managing a meal plan	Compassionate things I can say to myself or do to help me manage my meal plan
I don't like to plan when and what to eat.	*Most people don't like to plan like this. But I deserve the opportunity to develop a better relationship with food. I have been able to schedule regular eating a little better. I can live with this for a while to see whether it can help me; if it doesn't, I can always stop doing it.*
Eating to a plan makes me feel controlled and brings up unhappy memories of the way people fed me in the past.	*It is really sad that people were controlled by eating in unhelpful and unkind ways in the past. It is also understandable, as overeating and dieting often helps you to feel in control. But now I am an adult I can choose to take control of my eating and learn new ways to take control of my life. I don't really control food anyway; it controls me because I can't stop overeating when I want to.*
I don't know what a normal portion of pizza is.	*I can look up what a normal portion is in my calorie-counting book. I can work out how many calories of pizza I am going to eat as part of my evening meal and allow myself this.*
The plan does not give me any freedom.	*If I give myself too much freedom, I know I will overeat. It is worth having some constraints to help me work out why I overeat. I can choose what I eat on the plan.*
It's hard to keep to the plan when other people are around.	*Everyone struggles to eat consistently when they are with others. I can plan in advance for the kind of meal other people might eat. I can use this as a chance to practise saying no when people offer me food.*

Meal planning is a 'live and learn' process, and we're all likely to come up against a number of challenges as we go. No one's expecting you to keep to your meal plan all of the time; that would be unrealistic for any of us! The key is to stick to it as much as possible. That way it can serve its purpose as a way of retraining your body to eat what it needs and when it needs to eat it, and to help you identify the various influences that lead to overeating so you can work on them.

Step 3: Balancing your energy needs

The first thing to do in drawing up a meal plan is to work out your energy needs and match this with your food intake, so that you are eating approximately the amount of calories your body is going to use up. However, first a word of caution: there's quite a high risk that putting this step into action may trigger your dieting mindset. If your overeating has led to weight gain, you're likely to lose some weight as you establish a better energy balance. It's all too easy to become fixed on this as an achievement in itself, or to become impatient with the rate of loss and try to eat less than our bodies need. Also, if we try to reduce our overeating too rapidly, we run the risk of triggering our famine survival responses, as described in Chapter 2. So here are some guidelines to help you manage this step:

1. Know what your needs are now.

2. Know by how much you are overeating or undereating.

3. Don't reduce your energy intake too quickly.

4. Plan your eating at least one day in advance.

Know what your needs are now

We explored our energy and nutritional needs in some detail in Chapter 13. You can use this information as the basis of your meal plan.

Know by how much you are overeating or undereating

Again, the information you collected in Chapter 13 will help you to calculate this. Remember to look at these needs day to day as well as across the week, to avoid the urge to overeat that comes from trying to 'make up' for overeating on the previous day.

Don't reduce your intake too quickly

Most of us will be familiar with the notion that diets would only aim to reduce our weight by 1–2 lb (0.5–1 kg) a week. The evidence suggests that this is the most our body can manage healthily. If you tend to overeat as a consequence of getting caught up in a dieting mindset when you start to reduce the amount you're eating, even this may be too much. Ideally, you might aim to reduce your overall energy intake by about 200 calories a day for one week, then the same the next week, until it roughly matches your daily energy needs and you are in a neutral energy balance. Remember, changing your eating is a long-term process, and the goal is to make changes that will last. This becomes a little easier if we make smaller, but sustainable, changes in our eating.

Plan your eating at least one day in advance

This does require some forward thinking, and you may find it difficult at first; but over time you will get used to having a range of options of foods you enjoy and that meet your energy needs so that you can ring the changes from day to day, without having to start from scratch every time. The principles of drawing up a meal plan are basically the same as those you used to establish a regular eating pattern in the previous chapter, and you can use a similar form to set out your plan. This is provided in Worksheet 20. The only differences are that now you are planning what types of food (to help you develop a healthy nutritional balance) and how much you will eat (so you can roughly balance your eating intake with your energy needs). The comments section is there for you to write down any difficulties you have had following your plan and ways you have addressed or could address them in future. I have provided a worksheet for a seven-episode eating plan. The number of episodes will depend on how long you are awake. I suggest a minimum of five episodes per day. If you have fewer episodes, you will need more food at each one.

So, meal planning has the same five rules as for planning regular eating, with two new ones added:

1. Plan when you are going to eat.

2. Plan how much food you are going to eat at each episode.

3. Eat by the clock, not your feelings.

4. Eat every three to four hours.

5. Do not skip an eating episode.

6. Do not add an eating episode.

7. Drink enough fluid (about eight glasses, or 2 litres) a day.

In Figure 15.2 you will find a sample day's meal plan to guide you.

Worksheet 20: Tomorrow's meal plan

Meal or snack	Time and place, and who with	Food and drink to be taken, including type and amount	Comments (Including any problems in keeping to my plan, any solutions for these problems or changes to the plan)
Breakfast			
Mid-morning snack			
Lunch			

Mid-afternoon snack	Evening meal	Evening snack	Supper

Figure 15.2 Alison's meal plan

Meal or snack	Time and place, and who with	Food and drink to be taken, including type and amount	Comments (Including any problems in keeping to my plan, any solutions for these problems or changes to the plan)
Breakfast	7.30 a.m. At home, alone	STARCH – 1 bowl of cereal, 2 slices of toast FAT – butter SUGAR – jam FLUID – 1 cup of tea	
Mid-morning snack	10.30 a.m. At work at my desk, with colleagues	DAIRY – 1 non-diet yoghurt FRUIT – 1 apple FLUID – 1 coffee	
Lunch	1 p.m. Office canteen, with colleagues	STARCH – medium-sized baked potato FAT – mayonnaise PROTEIN – 1 small tin of baked beans	

		VEG – side salad DAIRY – 2 scoops of ice cream FLUID – 1 glass of water
Mid-afternoon snack	4.30 p.m. At my desk, with colleagues	FRUIT – 1 banana (and fruit juice) FLUID – small glass of fruit juice
Evening meal	8 p.m. At home, alone	STARCH – 4 heaped tablespoons of rice FAT – cooking oil PROTEIN – stir-fried salmon VEG – stir-fry vegetables SUGAR – 1 chocolate-covered biscuit FLUID – 1 glass of squash
Evening snack	No snack due to late evening meal	FLUID – 1 cup of decaffeinated coffee at 10 p.m.
Supper	11 p.m. At home with partner	DAIRY – 1 cup of warm milk

Step 4: Developing a healthy nutritional balance

Sometimes when we begin to plan our meals, we can also begin to change the types of food we eat. However, many of us find this a step too far at first, which is why Step 3 simply concentrated on planning how much and when you will eat. Once you have established your meal plan, however, and are getting used to aiming at a neutral energy balance, you can work at getting a better nutritional balance as well. You can use the information in Chapter 13 (especially figures 13.1 and 13.2) to guide you on proportions of the various food types. One of the problems that can arise with doing this is that we are often brought up to associate healthy eating with boring meals or feeling forced to eat foods we don't like. The key to improving our nutritional balance is to explore and experiment with a wider range of foods. For example, you might think you don't like the taste of vegetables – but there are an awful lot of different vegetables, and maybe you were put off by just one or two, perhaps always cooked the same way. So, you may need to try a lot of different types, cooked and prepared in quite a lot of ways, before you can really decide what you like.

This can be quite an exciting time in your process of tackling overeating. Here are a few tips you might want to try to help you:

- Use your meal plan and the information in Chapter 13 to explore how your current eating fits with a nutritionally balance food intake.

- Try to make small changes in your balance and then build on them. For example, you may want to increase your intake of fruit and vegetables by 100 calories a day at first, swapping this number of calories for another food type (perhaps reducing sugary or higher-fat foods by the same amount).

- Have some fun experimenting with food. For example, you might write the names of twenty types of fruit on pieces of paper, mix them up and pick one at random. Go and find one of whatever it is. If you really don't like it, try something else.

- Experiment with cooking food as well. For example, my kids really don't like carrot that much, so my wife mashes it with potato.

- Learn what you like and don't like; and don't eat what you don't like!

Step 5: Learning to respond to feelings of hunger and fullness

Meal planning is designed to help us retrain our eating patterns so that we can then move on to deciding what and when to eat on the basis of whether our body feels hungry or full, rather than on the basis of our habits and emotions. Within the structure of regular, balanced eating that your meal plans provide, you will gradually learn to experience these feelings of hunger and fullness. A healthier nutritional balance will mean that most of the calories we eat come from the types of food that are most likely to help us feel full and satisfied.

Some diets will have trained your body to respond to fluid as if it were food, for example by getting you to drink a lot before you eat. A recent study has shown that this doesn't really work that well at a biological level, as our body recognises the energy content of food, not simply the volume in our stomachs. However, drinking too much before you eat can make it more difficult for you to work out whether you are full or not, so at first you may find it easier to drink when you have finished eating.

Often the ways in which we eat can obscure our natural feelings of hunger or fullness or lead us to ignore our body's signals. To become aware of them again we may need to learn to be more mindful of the experience of eating. If we think about which Western countries have the longest lifespan and most healthy lifestyles, we tend to think of the countries of southern Europe and the 'Mediterranean diet'. This is based around fresh fruit and vegetables, starchy food such as pasta, and protein from meat and fish.

However, this is only part of the story. The Mediterranean diet is also associated with a very specific way of eating. Eating tends to be a shared family ritual, each dish is savoured, and a meal can last for several hours – including the occasional glass of wine, also sipped and savoured rather than gulped down. This is in fact the very type of eating we evolved for. The key point is that food is not just fuel that we eat in front of the TV, at our desks or work-stations, or even behind the steering wheel. Allowing ourselves to eat more slowly, to savour the tastes and textures of food, and to begin to digest one course before we decide whether we want the next one, can all help us listen to our body and become more sensitive to its signals.

You can add this step at any stage of your journey to a new way of eating. However, the reason I have put it here, towards the end of the six-step programme, is that if your eating has become entangled with managing difficult feelings, then being more in touch with feelings of hunger and fullness may also put you in touch with difficult emotional experiences or memories. If this is the case for you, it can be helpful to eat in a less mindful way in the early stages of changing your eating. Nevertheless, to beat overeating for good we do need to become more mindful when we are eating or when we have the urge to eat. You can use your eating diary to help you note down any thoughts and feelings that you have when you eat more mindfully.

If you feel ready to embark on this step, start by becoming more mindful of the physical experience of hunger, so you can begin to use this as a guide to when to eat and how much you need. Sometimes it is easier to recognise when we have eaten far too much than when we are hungry. So, to begin with, spend a little time remembering the last time this happened:

- How did your body feel?

- When did you notice that you had eaten too much?

- What happened that helped you to ignore these feelings of becoming full while you were still eating?

Next you may want to think about the last time you were so extremely hungry that you found it really hard to stop eating once you had started:

- How did this feel in your body?

- What things had led you to ignore your hunger this much?

Finally, think about the last time you felt you had eaten just enough to feel satisfied (a bit like Goldilocks and her porridge – you got it just right!). This is the sensation that you want to experience to guide you in knowing when your body has had enough to eat. Sometimes we will not get this absolutely right – we will have eaten just a little too much or remain just a bit hungry.

Try to bring to mind each of these stages and explore how it felt and what helped you to notice when you had eaten enough or just slightly more than your body needed. You can practise this skill by rating your hunger and fullness, and we will explore this in the next exercise.

Exercise 15.2: Learning to feel hunger and fullness

In this exercise you can work on becoming more mindful of your body's hunger and fullness signals. To begin with, make a note every time you eat of how hungry you feel before and how full you feel after. You could do this in your eating diary or meal plan if you're still keeping one. When you have a better idea, you can move on to the next stage, which is to track these sensations during the day, and when you are actually eating. As you develop this skill, you can then use the knowledge you gain to decide when you need to eat and when you have had enough. It can also be helpful to make a note of whether other things interfere with your ability to keep an eye on (and respond to) your body's needs – for example, feeling tired, angry or upset, or becoming too engrossed in other activities.

You can use the following rating scales to help you. The 'hungriness scale' is something you can use throughout the day, perhaps keeping a note of your score every hour or so and every time you eat. If you use it together with your eating diary it can help you to explore any things that increase your hunger. These may include a desire to eat that is triggered by changes in your blood sugar levels when you need food; however, you may also notice associations between certain feelings (such as tiredness or anger) and increased feelings of hunger. The 'fullness scale' is designed to be used while you are eating, so perhaps just keep a note of changes in feelings of fullness during your meal and for around thirty minutes after you finish.

Hungriness scale:

1 = Extremely hungry – so much so that you will find it very hard to stop eating when you are full or that you can't wait for your next meal.

2 = Moderately hungry – you may still be inclined to overeat or to snack a little before your next meal.

3 = Slightly hungry – you may have strong urges to overeat or snack and have to work hard to resist.

4 = Ready to eat – you know you are ready for your next meal but don't have a strong urge to snack and are unlikely to overeat when you have it.

5 = Don't need to eat – you don't feel hungry and if you were to eat now you would feel overfull.

Fullness scale:

1 = Not full at all – you are still hungry after your meal and are very likely to overeat.

2 = Moderately full – you are still a bit hungry and want to carry on eating; you may end up overeating.

3 = Full and satisfied – you have eaten enough to feel full and don't want to eat any more.

4 = Overfull – you have eaten more than enough, perhaps eating a few bites more than you need.

5 = Far too full – you feel very uncomfortable with the amount you have eaten, perhaps bloated, even physically unwell.

Ideally, we want to start eating as soon as we start feeling hungry (4 on the hungriness scale) and stop when we reach 3 on the fullness scale, so that we will not overeat. You may need to spend some time learning to do this, as we can all get a little out of touch with our body's needs; the key is to try to avoid getting so detached from what your body is telling you that you end up getting very hungry and then overeating as a result. It is also important to remember that your body tends to take a little while to give you signals that you are full; so, eating more slowly with fewer distractions is really important at this stage, so that you can become aware of feelings of fullness gradually growing.

What am I hungry for?

I had a discussion with a dietitian colleague of mine who regularly asks her clients an interesting question in relation to eating more mindfully: 'What are you hungry for?' Now, as a psychologist, I thought she meant: *What emotional needs is your eating helping you with?* – an important aspect of this work. However, this wasn't quite what she had meant. She was interested in our body's intuitive wisdom in knowing what it needs and hungering for that thing in order to feel satisfied. The most extreme example of this can be some of the curious food cravings that happen during pregnancy. But let's take a more everyday example. Imagine you really want some orange-flavoured chocolate but deny yourself this and have an orange instead. My guess is that no matter how many oranges you eat you will still be 'hungry' for the chocolate. Being aware of this can help you to recognise what it is you want and then be satisfied with a little of it, rather than spending so much time denying your needs that you eat food you don't want and then, having denied yourself and so increased the craving, end up overeating the thing you wanted in the first place!

Step 6: Learning to enjoy food again

This is your final step along the road to a new way of eating. By this stage you should be able to keep (mostly) to your meal plans and be more in touch with your body's needs. You will also be able to recognise trigger foods and other things that are likely to lead to overeating.

You may also have included in your planned eating some of the foods that you enjoy. However, some foods that you used to enjoy may now have less pleasant associations – you may like the taste of cakes but have learned to be afraid of the consequences of eating them. Or you may have always eaten sweets when you overate but ate so many so fast that you never really knew whether you liked the taste. You may have eaten so much of a particular food that all you associate with it now is the experience of feeling overfull and bloated.

If certain foods have specific unpleasant associations for you, you may wish to start to weaken and break these links so that you can once again allow yourself to enjoy them. The next exercise can help you do this.

Exercise 15.3: Changing food associations

Choose a food that you have previously been concerned about eating but think that you might enjoy or would like to eat again. Plan to eat some of this food at a time you do not feel hungry. Then bring your soothing system into play. When you feel ready, put a piece of the food in your mouth. Take time to experience the smell, taste and texture of the food, and try to answer the following questions:

- What do you notice?

- Is the food something that you like?

- Does eating the food trigger any other experiences – for example, unpleasant memories?

- What might worry you if you allowed yourself to enjoy what you have eaten?

If you notice memories, thoughts and feelings rising up that could stop you enjoying the food, don't eat any more just now but pause and write these down. Now think what your compassionate mind might say or do to help you cope with these thoughts. You could use a version of Worksheet 7, or you might like to write yourself a compassionate letter to help you.

When you feel ready, you can repeat the exercise with another piece of the food; but this time, gently and kindly, imagine – or even actually say out loud – these compassionate thoughts as you are eating. With practice you will learn to associate these new thoughts with these foods and to allow yourself to enjoy them. As well as returning to foods you used to enjoy, try to increase the variety that you eat so you can learn that you enjoy exploring new tastes, smells and textures.

Another aspect of learning to enjoy food again is getting used to eating with others. Many people who overeat have come to avoid eating socially, either because they are concerned what other people might think about what they eat (for example, seeing them as greedy) or because they are more likely to overeat in these situations. Again, this is something you can overcome with practice – after all, you deserve to eat out, and to eat with your friends and family, as much as anyone else! This is the time to learn to reclaim eating as a pleasant and normal human social activity that you no longer need to be afraid of. The next exercise will help you to do this.

Exercise 15.4: Enjoying eating socially

Again, you can use Worksheet 7 to help you. Begin by writing down in the left-hand column any thoughts or feelings that have stopped you, or put you off, eating with other people. Now bring your compassionate mind into play and explore ways in which you could address these concerns from a compassionate perspective. If you have noted that you are concerned about how other people would react to seeing you eat, you might want to think about this from the perspective of your compassionate image; would they see it as fair to stop people eating socially and enjoying food?

Another way to begin feeling more comfortable eating socially is gradually to build up the range of people you eat with or places where you eat. For example, you might start by having a meal with just one other person you know, like and trust, and then try eating with a small group of two or three people. This will give you the opportunity to practise your new compassionate thoughts and behaviour. When you feel comfortable, you could then gradually expand the range of people you eat with and places where you eat.

The key to this last step in the programme is to experiment and learn to have fun with foods. Allow yourself to reclaim your relationship with eating, so that you enjoy food, safe in the knowledge that you are in tune with your body's needs and have alternative ways of managing your feelings. It is this feeling of pleasure and safety, rather than the rigid (and impossible) rules of dieting, or the chaos of overeating to manage your feelings or from habit, which will make eating a 'risk free' and enjoyable part of your life.

Putting it all together: caring for your body with compassion

Our bodies need to be cared for if we are going to get the most out of them, and eating healthily is a big part of this – but it is not the whole story. None of us is going to have the perfect body! A more realistic aim is to have a body that is healthy for as long as possible, and that we appreciate and enjoy. To achieve this, we need not only to eat well, but also to attend to two of our other needs: *activity* and *rest*.

Physical activity

Our long-term health has far more to do with how physically fit we are than how much we weigh. The good news is that our bodies are relatively low maintenance compared to those of a thoroughbred racehorse (or even our pet dogs). We need about one hour of physical activity every day that increases out heart rate and keeps it up, without making us out of breath (a good indicator of this is whether we can still keep up a conversation). It seems that we can even do this in short bursts of five to ten minutes and still get the same health benefits. Sadly, most of us – including me! – don't always do this. We tend to be very sedentary, because of the changes in lifestyle that have come with working longer and longer hours in less physical jobs. Or we engage in intense programmes of activity that we find hard to sustain – typically as a New Year's resolution to join a gym.

Our average levels of physical activity, particularly among younger people, are going down year by year. For a whole range of reasons, people who overeat tend to do even less physical activity than the already unhealthily low average. This is not good for our mental or our physical health. Lack of activity can lead to low mood, tiredness and anxiety, and a range of physical problems, as well as leaving us weighing more than our genetic make-up intended.

However, many of us also over-exercise, usually by setting targets that are not sustainable – for example, vowing that we will go running every day, come rain or shine. We also tend to link exercise with the dieting mindset: we exercise to lose weight and give it up when we give up our diet.

So, we need to aim for a compassionate level of physical activity that recognises and is in tune with our body's needs, but that also reflects and responds to our physical health – so that, for example, we don't force ourselves to go running when we are ill. We also need to break the link between 'exercise' and the dieting mindset. In fact, it can be better not to think of 'exercise' at all, but of 'physical activity' instead. For many of us, formal exercise can have a whole range of negative connections – for example, with being bullied into cross-country running at school, or being humiliated by not being picked for the football or hockey team. For others, exercise simply became 'uncool' and was abandoned as they grew older.

Starting formal exercise or taking up sport again can take a lot of courage if we've had any of these types of experience in the past – and it can be even harder if we don't feel good about our fitness levels or our size and shape. Many people can and do find going to the gym or taking up a sport a fun and useful way to increase their physical activity. However, physical activity covers a whole range of things a long way from gym workouts and exercise classes. It can include dancing around at home, going for a walk, gardening – even housework.

The key to increasing it is to choose a variety of things you're prepared to do now, and a couple you'd like to work towards. Remember, variety is the spice of life; an extra hour of housework may increase your activity levels but may not be as much fun as going for a walk with a friend!

Increasing your physical activity will take some planning, and you might want to add it in to your meal planning. If you do this, you can use your increased activity to improve your energy balance – but do bear in mind that activity tends to make us hungry, so we need to plan to eat and replace fluid afterwards.

Start by increasing your levels slowly: listen to your body and ease off when it tells you that you're doing too much. Remember, you should still be able to hold a conversation; pushing through pain is not necessary and it's certainly not compassionate. The usual advice also applies before you begin to increase your activity – check with your doctor that there's no medical reason why you shouldn't.

If you are taking at least an hour's physical activity a day, then you are meeting your body's needs. Anything over and above this will affect your energy balance for the day. As you get more in touch with your hunger you are likely to notice this increase in energy need, and to respond to it appropriately.

Rest

Our body needs time to rest and repair itself just as much as it needs food to fuel it and physical activity to maintain it. We get most of the rest we need when we sleep, but we also need to have some during the day, particularly if we have just finished physical activity (and more than usual, of course, if we are unwell).

It is easy to work all day, come home and do housework and look after other people, or even carry on working from home, right up until bedtime. If we don't get enough rest, we can end up feeling stressed, anxious, depressed and irritable – all of which can lead to overeating. So, we may need to plan in periods of rest during the day, even if it is only a couple of minutes at a time. This can also help us to learn why we don't allow ourselves to rest. It may be that we have simply got out of the habit; but it may also be that we keep busy to avoid difficult thoughts and feelings, or because we feel compelled to. You might like to use some of the exercises in Chapter 7 to help you explore and overcome these obstacles to taking rest.

Many people who overeat also have problems with sleeping. Lack of sleep can directly increase our likelihood of overeating. If we are awake for longer periods we have more opportunities for overeating; not having enough sleep also lowers our mood and leaves us too tired to plan our eating and prepare food, or to keep physically active. It can even leave us craving foods to give us an energy burst – usually those high in fat and sugar! Sleep problems can be a complicated area. However, the following simple 'sleep hygiene' tips can help:

- Always get up at the same time, no matter how tired you are.

- Don't sleep during the day.

- Only go to bed when you are tired.

- Use your bed for sleeping, don't sleep elsewhere, e.g. in a chair or on the sofa.

You may wish to develop a bedtime routine to prepare you for sleep. This could usefully include the following strategies:

- Cut out caffeinated drinks (coffee, tea, cola, etc.) for at least four hours before bedtime.

- Avoid drinking alcohol for a couple of hours before going to bed.

- Don't overstimulate your mind by doing mentally challenging work, playing computer games, or watching scary or upsetting TV programmes for a couple of hours before bedtime.

- Have a milky drink before you go to bed.

- Spend a little time getting ready for bed, getting changed into your nightclothes, cleaning your teeth etc., to give yourself the message that you are going to sleep soon.

- If you like to read in bed, try to choose something that is not too interesting or emotionally stimulating.

- If you can't sleep after ten minutes, get up and repeat your bedtime ritual until you feel sleepy.

This type of sleeping plan may well leave you feeling exhausted for a week or two but can be very effective in establishing a sleep routine. We all struggle to get to sleep, or to stay asleep, at times in our lives, but usually this phase passes after a day or two. If you have problems with sleeping that last longer than this, have a word with your doctor. In the further reading section for this chapter, you can also find details of a book that will help you work on this on your own.

My personal reflections on Chapter 15

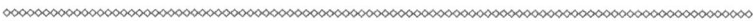

You might find it helpful to write down your key personal learning points from this chapter.

- What blocks to meal planning have you encountered and how have you addressed them?

- What has it been like to learn to enjoy eating again?

- What long-term commitments to increasing your levels of activity and improving rest have you made?

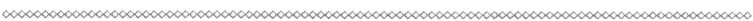

SUMMARY

This chapter has taken you through the final steps towards a new way of eating. These include planning your energy balance and nutritional needs, learning to respond to natural feelings of hunger and fullness, and learning to enjoy food again, both on your own and in company. We've also explored how to care for your body in other ways by getting appropriate amounts of activity and rest.

It may be that these practical approaches are enough to help you to stop overeating, or at least to improve how often it happens and how severe it gets. However much we plan, though, our emotions and thoughts can still get in the way and may still trigger overeating from time to time, even when we have established a better structure to our eating, and you are likely to need the skills and wisdom you have been developing throughout the book to help you with this. The final chapter summarises how to do this.

16 A compassionate approach to eating well – some final thoughts

This final chapter will bring together some of the ideas that have run through the whole book. To begin with, here are ten key reminders:

1. Our relationship with food and eating can be very complicated. We evolved with a 'see-food-and-eat-it' brain and body, and an emotional system to help us survive in a world full of threats. We did not evolve for a sedentary lifestyle in a world of plenty with a powerful food industry that has created a huge range of easily accessible and highly appetising foods, many of which are high in fat and sugar. We are now subject to far fewer direct physical threats, but our stressed emotional systems can become very entangled with our eating.

2. A desire to overeat, therefore, is *absolutely not your fault* but the result of a whole range of factors, many of which we have no control over. So, no matter what you weigh or what you eat there's nothing to be ashamed about – no matter what society says: remember, in some societies plumpness is a sign of beauty and wealth! However, how you eat and care for your body more generally *is your responsibility* – and you can learn to look after yourself in new ways that are better for your physical and emotional health than relying on overeating to cope.

3. Learning to be compassionate – kindly and more relaxed about your eating, rather than anxious, depressed and self-critical – can be the first step on a journey towards these new ways of eating and taking responsibility for yourself.

4. Learning why compassion is so beneficial for you, for example by understanding the 'three systems' model of our emotions, will help you to see the value of living more compassionately. Remember, compassion is not about being soft or self-indulgent, or about letting our guard down. It's about developing a very important inner quality, related to how our brain works, that will help us face difficulties in our lives, and cope with setbacks and disappointments.

5. Learning to become more aware – more *mindful* – of the urges to eat and the act of eating, and then of the link between our emotions and our eating, is a key step. This book has given you many ideas for exploring how to become more aware of when, what and why you eat what you do. It will help you understand how eating might have come to have emotional significance for you, for example as a comfort eater.

6. Understanding your personal history, in terms of how your eating styles have evolved over time, can be especially useful. You may want to explore these ideas again from time to time. Different things may occur to you at different points on your journey, and as you move on you may gain different insights into your personal history and its links to your overeating.

7. Developing and understanding of your personal relationship with food can help you to come up with new ways of dealing with food and your feelings – not in an aggressive, forceful way but in a compassionate way, using your wisdom, courage and dedication to make long-term changes.

8. Learning to stand back from setbacks, and being open, curious and compassionate about them, can help you understand what they were about, what triggered them, and how you might respond differently next time. Getting angry with yourself, or becoming depressed, when setbacks occur is only likely to lead to further episodes of overeating.

9. Taking practical steps such as meal planning, choosing healthy eating, and gradually switching from unhealthy foods to more healthy ones will help to change your relationship with food (for example, stopping buying foods you know tend to trigger overeating for you). These steps allow you to gradually learn to trust your body's responses to eating, for example its natural signals of hunger and fullness, and to begin to enjoy eating again.

10. Developing your compassionate mind, for example through imagery exercises, will strengthen your capacity for compassion, both towards yourself and towards others. In working through this book, you have learned how to develop your soothing system, manage difficult emotional experiences and tolerate and mindfully explore your feelings. The key principle underlying all these changes is the development of a compassionate approach to eating well and caring for your body's needs for activity and rest. In all kinds of situations from now on, you can ask yourself, 'What would compassionate attention be focused on here? What would compassionate thinking be in this situation? How can I behave compassionately to myself or others in these circumstances? If I take a breath and slow down, and switch on my compassionate mind, how would it help me?' Compassionate letter writing can be a great help in dealing with the challenges that lie ahead. You can also use it to plan more things that are fun

and exciting in your life (developing your drive system) and allow yourself to experience more joy from being in your soothing system, whether on your own or with other people.

There are a lot of ideas in this book – you may even feel that there are too many, or that the prospect of change is too complex, difficult or overwhelming. The key is to try things out for yourself and see what you can use. Few of us follow manuals or recipes to the letter, but we also know that if we want to learn to drive, play a musical instrument or speak Spanish, the more we practise the better we'll get. If you think (as many of us will) 'This can't work for me', you can bring your compassionate mind online and let it wonder why you might say this. You can then see this concern as an interesting question rather than a definitive statement. Perhaps you can allow your compassionate mind to gently support and encourage you and say, 'Maybe this will work for me; let me give it a try to find out if it can.' Remember, your threat system may be used to running your life and may be very worried about change!

Don't be frightened of asking for help, either: there are increasing numbers of dietitians and organisations you can consult. Sometimes your family doctor can be very helpful in advising you on what is available locally. Many people find that having the support of others is really valuable – although keep in mind that diet groups that focus too much on weight loss, rather than healthy eating and healthy living, may not be such a good idea, particularly if you find that your 'dieting mindset' leads to overeating (and longer-term weight gain). Nonetheless, sharing your thoughts and experiences with others, and feeling supported and understood by them, can be very helpful, and seeking support is a very compassionate thing to do. If you would like some guidelines on where to look, try the 'Useful resources' section at the end of this book. If you prefer not to meet others in person, there are also options for making contact on the internet or over the phone. The resources section also contains information on where you can find help in becoming more self-compassionate, and in working on overeating. Take your time to explore the possibilities and use your compassionate wisdom to help you decide which ones are likely to be most helpful to you.

I hope that the approach set out in this book will help you learn to change unhelpful eating habits and enable you to enjoy the wonderful tastes, textures and smells of food, and the opportunity to share these with people you care about and who care for you. I hope that it helps you find a better relationship with physical activity, rest and your overall emotional wellbeing. I hope you find ways to experience the fun and sense of achievement your drive offers, and joy and contentment from your soothing system. All of these are important elements of the compassionate approach to eating well.

All that remains for me to do is to send you many compassionate best wishes in your new and developing relationship with food and your body. As they say in compassionate practice:

May you be well.

May you be happy.

May you be free from suffering.

And may compassionate eating be an integral part of your life.

Appendix 1: Useful resources

Compassion

The Compassionate Mind Foundation (www.compassionatemind.co.uk)

In 2007, Paul Gilbert and a number of colleagues (including myself) set up a charity called The Compassionate Mind Foundation. On its website, you'll find various essays and details of other sites that look at different aspects of compassion. The charity also offers training and a 'find a therapist/supervisor' service.

Balanced Minds (balancedminds.com)

This is a UK organisation that provides world-class psychological services and resources. It offers in person and online therapy, training, coaching, supervision, training workshops, consultation and help to improve workplace wellbeing.

Mind and Life Institute (www.mindandlife.org)

The Dalai Lama has formed relationships with Western scientists to develop a more compassionate way of living. More information on this can be found on this website.

The Center for Compassion and Altruism Research and Education (ccare.stanford.edu)

The website of an institution set up to promote and support international work on the advancement of compassion.

Self-compassion (self-compassion.org)

This website is run by one of the leading researchers on self-compassion.

Eating disorders and overeating

The Eating Well Workbook: A Compassion Focused, Therapist-guided Self-help Intervention for Clients Who Overeat

This workbook is designed for compassion focused therapists to use in conjunction with this book, to provide additional support for people who overeat. It can be found online at overcoming. co.uk/715/resources-to-download.

BEAT (www.beateatingdisorders.org.uk)

BEAT is the UK's leading eating disorders charity, offering of helpful information and support for people with eating disorders and disordered eating.

Academy for Eating Disorders (AED) (www.aedweb.org)

This website is aimed mainly at professionals working with people with eating disorders, but it is also a good source of information for the public.

National Eating Disorder Information Centre (www.nedic.ca)

This Canadian non-profit organisation provides information and resources on eating disorders and preoccupations with food and weight.

Lindo Bacon (https://lindobacon.com/_resources/haes-contributions)

This non-dieting approach to eating and health is becoming increasingly popular. This website contains useful articles and downloads for individuals and healthcare providers.

Compassion focused therapy and eating disorders/eating distress

Gale, C., Gilbert, P., Read, N. and Goss, K. (2012) 'An evaluation of the impact of introducing compassion focused therapy to a standard treatment programme for people with eating disorders', *Clinical Psychology and Psychotherapy*, 21, 1–12.

Goss, K. and Allan, A. (2010) 'Compassion focused therapy for eating disorders', *International Journal of Cognitive Therapy*, 3, 141–58.

Goss, K. and Allan, S. (2012) 'An introduction to compassion focused therapy for eating disorders', In J. Fox and K. Goss (eds), *Eating and Its Disorders* (pp. 303–15). New Jersey, NJ: Wiley-Blackwell.

Goss, K. and Allan, S. (2014) 'The development and application of compassion-focused therapy for eating disorders (CFT-E)', *British Journal of Clinical Psychology*, 53, 62–77.

Goss, K. and Gilbert, P. (2002) 'Eating disorders, shame and pride: a cognitive–behavioural functional analysis', In P. Gilbert and J. Miles (eds), *Body Shame: Conceptualisation, Research and Treatment* (pp. 219–55). London: Brunner-Routledge.

Goss, K. and Haynes, C. (2022) 'Compassion focused therapy for people with an eating disorder', In J. Downs, M. Hopfenbeck, H. Lewis, I. Parker and N. Schanckenberg (eds), *The Practical Handbook of Eating Difficulties: A Comprehensive Guide from Personal and Professional Perspectives* (pp. 255–64). West Sussex: Pavilion.

Goss, K. and Kelly, A. (2022) 'The role of shame, self-criticism and compassion focused therapy in eating disorders and disordered eating', In P. Gilbert and G. Simos (eds), *Compassion Focused Therapy: Clinical Practice and Applications* (pp. 519–33). Oxfordshire: Routledge.

Harris, R.B.S. (1990) 'Role of set point theory in regulation of body weight', *FASEB Journal,* 4(15), 3310–3318. doi.org/10.1096/fasebj.4.15.225384

Marques, C.C. Palmeira, L., Castilho, P., Rodrigues, D., Mayr, A., Pina, T.S., Pereira, A.T., Castelo-Branco, M. and Goss, K. (2024) 'Online compassion focused therapy for overeating: feasibility and acceptability pilot study', *International Journal of Eating Disorders,* 57(2), 410–22. doi.org/10.1002/eat.24118

Steindl, S., Buchanan, K., Goss, K. and Allan, S. (2017) 'Compassion focused therapy for eating disorders: a qualitative review and recommendations for further applications', *Clinical Psychologist,* 21(2), 62–73. doi.org/10.1111/cp.12126

Vrabel, K.R., Wampold, B., Quintana, D.S., Goss, K., Waller, G. and Hoffart, A. (2019) 'The Modum-ED trial protocol: comparing compassion-focused therapy and cognitive-behavioral therapy in treatment of eating disorders with and without childhood trauma: protocol of a randomized trial', *Frontiers of Psychology,* 18(10), 1638. doi.10.3389/fpsyg.2019.01638

Vrabel, K.R., Wampold, B., Quintana, D.S., Goss, K., Waller, G. and Hoffart, A. (2024) 'Cognitive behavioral therapy versus compassion focused therapy for adult patients with eating disorders with and without childhood trauma: a randomized controlled trial in an intensive treatment setting', *Behaviour Research and Therapy,* 174, 104480. doi: 10.1016/j.brat.2024.104480

Appendix 2: Further reading

Chapter 2: Making sense of overeating, part 1 – how our bodies work

On maintenance of weight loss: National Heart, Lung and Blood Institute Obesity Education and Innovation Expert Panel (1998) 'Clinical guidelines on the identification, evaluation and treatment of overweight and obesity in adults: the evidence report', *Obesity Research*, 6, 51S–209S.

On blood sugar levels and appetite: *Logue, A.W. (2004)* The Psychology of Eating and Drinking, *3rd edn. New York: Brunner-Routledge, p. 182.*

On the starve–eat cycle: Keys, A., Broze, J. and Henschel, A. (1950) *The Biology of Human Starvation*, Vol. 2. Minneapolis: Minnesota University Press.

On the body's natural tendency to increase physical activity to match increased energy intake: Levine, J.A., Ebhardt, N.L. and Jensen, M.D. (1999) 'Role of nonexercise activity thermogenesis in resistance to fat gain in humans', *Science*, 283, 212–214.

Chapter 3: Making sense of overeating, part 2 – eating and our feelings

On how we learn to eat: Booth, D.A. (1994) *The Psychology of Nutrition*. London: Taylor & Francis. Provides a fascinating review of how we learn to eat, how our eating patterns change as we grow older, and the psychological and biological influences on eating.

On emotional and hormonal fluctuations in adolescence: A good overview of this fascinating stage in our development, and the challenges it can present, can be found at http://en.wikipedia.org/wiki/Adolescence.

On the threat system of emotional regulation: Baumeister, R.F., Bratslavsky, E., Finkenauer, C. and Vohs, K.D. (2001) 'Bad is stronger than good', *Review of General Psychology*, 5, 323–70.

On the areas of our brain and hormones that respond to kindness: *See references in Gilbert, P. (2009)* The Compassionate Mind. *London: Robinson, Chapter 5.*

On the psychological distress experienced by people coming to NHS weight loss services: Webb, C. (2000) 'Psychological distress in clinical obesity: the role of eating disorder beliefs and behaviours, social comparison and shame'. Unpublished doctoral manuscript, University of Leicester.

Chapter 4: The compassionate mind

For a detailed overview of the compassion focused approach, see *Gilbert, P. (2009) The Compassionate Mind. London: Robinson.*

Chapter 12: Compassionately motivating *yourself* to change

On psychological research on change: Prochaska, J.W. and DiClemente, C.C. (1983) 'Stages and processes of self-change of smoking: toward an integrative model of change', *Journal of Consulting and Clinical Psychology*, 51(3), 390–95.

Chapter 15: Towards a new way of eating – the final steps

On establishing a sleep routine: For more detailed help in managing sleep problems, see Espie, C. (2021) *Overcoming Insomnia*. London: Robinson.

Index

Note: page numbers in *italics* refer to worksheets, page numbers in **bold** refer to figures.